M000251637

Wound Care at End of Life
A Guide for Hospice Professionals
2nd edition

Joni Brinker, RN, MSN/MHA, WCC
Clinical Nurse Educator
Optum Hospice Pharmacy Services

Bridget McCrate Protus, PharmD, MLIS, BCGP, CDP
Director of Drug Information
Optum Hospice Pharmacy Services

Jason M. Kimbrel, PharmD, BCPS
Vice President of Operations & Clinical Services
Optum Hospice Pharmacy Services

Optum Hospice Pharmacy Services
4525 Executive Park Drive
Montgomery, AL 36166
Tel: 866-970-7500

Cover design: Scott J. McClusky

ISBN-13: 978-0-9889558-6-8

Acknowledgements
Kyna Setsor Shonkwiler, RN, BSN, CHPN
Content author for 1st edition; planning & development for 2nd edition
Optum Hospice Pharmacy Services

Melissa O'Neill Hunt, PharmD – Collaborator/Algorithm Design
Optum Hospice Pharmacy Services

Connie L. Bohn, RN, BSN, CWON
Content author & editor/reviewer for 1st edition

To the Staff of Optum Hospice Pharmacy Services
The authors wish to thank all of our colleagues for their assistance in the creation of this resource. Without their generous support this work would not have been possible. Their compassionate commitment to improving end of life care for all individuals is an inspiration.

This book provides guidance for the assessment and palliative management of wounds. Many factors influence whether healing a wound is a realistic goal. Whether the goal is for healing or for symptom relief, untreated wounds can lead to physical discomfort and impair quality of life. It is necessary that they receive appropriate intervention.

How to Use This Book
Wound Care at End of Life is a quick reference guide for palliative management of wounds in hospice care. The authors and collaborators have systematically reviewed and collected the pertinent literature and resources related to palliative wound care.

- For those already skilled in wound care, this book is a resource for support of current practices and a quick treatment lookup tool.
- For those with less wound care experience, this book can serve as a learning guide and resource to ensure best practices for palliative wound management.
- For educators, this book may be used as a training guide to address the basics of palliative wound care and assist learners in developing a comprehensive plan of care for the patient with wounds.

Table of Contents

INTRODUCTION TO PALLIATIVE WOUND CARE

Palliative care focuses on the holistic needs of an individual to promote comfort and quality of life in the face of an advanced disease process. This same focus applies to palliative wound care when patients with limited life expectancy have wounds that reduce their quality of life. Often, these wounds are an outward reflection of their inner disease process, can cause distressing symptoms, and may or may not heal. Thus, Tippett defined palliative wound care as the "the merging of symptom management into advanced wound care".[1] Certainly advanced wound care techniques are necessary to manage symptoms and complications of these wounds; however, in applying this definition, assess the appropriateness of wound care interventions in relation to the values of the patient, to the wound prognosis, and to the patient's life expectancy.[2] Ultimately, palliative wound care may use optimal wound treatment modalities, but emphasis is placed on the desires of the patient and the relief of symptoms, whether they are physical or psychological.[3] The result is an improved quality of life that allows patients and caregivers to focus on activities that are important to them.

References
1. Tippett A. An introduction to palliative chronic wound care. *Ostomy Wound Manage*. 2012;5:6-8.
2. Hughes RG, Bakos AD, O'Mara A, et al. Palliative wound care at the end of life. *Home Health Care Manag Pract*. 2005;17(3):196-202.
3. Hopkins HD. Psychological aspects of wound healing. *Nurs Times*. 2001;97(48):57.

GOALS OF CARE

"Comfort may be the overriding and acceptable goal, even though it may be in conflict with best skin care practice" Sibbald, Krasner, Lutz: SCALE[1]

Traditionally, wound goals of care reflect the desire to heal the wound by addressing the underlying disease process and providing appropriate topical dressings to promote growth of new tissue. Indicators of healing, such as the presence of granulation tissue or a decrease in wound size, demonstrate that the goal of care is achievable and the plan of care is appropriate. However, a comprehensive care plan for the palliative patient identifies patient-specific goals of care that reflect what is essential to improve quality of life for the patient.[2] For example, the goal of care for a palliative care patient with a pressure injury may be a reduction in the frequency of dressing changes or alleviation of distressing odor to improve

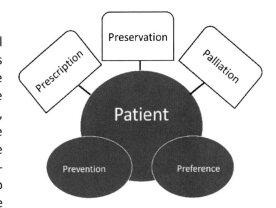

Figure 1. The 5 P's of Wound Care

quality of life. This does not mean that wound assessment or appropriate wound care practices are unnecessary. Wound assessments and advanced wound care techniques are still necessary to palliate symptoms and promote quality of life. Instead, use the assessment findings to identify possible prevention strategies and treatment options or constraints. Work with the patient and caregiver to develop a plan of care that is realistic and patient-centered. Subsequently, discuss the plan of care at each visit to encourage open lines of communication and ensure acceptable goals of care are in place.[1] The 5 P's assist in identifying the patient's preference, prevention strategies, and appropriate wound care goals and interventions (Figure 1):

Regardless of goal, PREVENTION and patient PREFERENCE are always included in the plan of care[1,3]
Prescription: Goal is wound healing with appropriate treatment. Care plan includes interventions for treatable wounds. Even at the end of life, some wounds may be healable with appropriate treatments. Interventions must: • Treat the cause • Remain patient-centered • Address quality of life concerns (e.g., pain, odor)
Preservation: Goal is stabilizing wound condition; healing is unlikely, but deterioration is preventable with appropriate treatment. Care plan recognizes that wound healing or improvement is limited; maintenance becomes the desired outcome. The wound may have the potential to heal, but overriding factors (e.g., the patient refuses treatment, caregiver limitations, inadequate nutrition) result in preservation as the care plan goal.
Palliation: Goal is comfort and symptom management; healing is not possible, and the wound may deteriorate even with best care. Care plan focuses on patient comfort, not healing, and acknowledges that wounds may deteriorate due to disease progression or dying process. Patients with palliative wound care goals may benefit from modest interventions (e.g., autolytic or enzymatic debridement, support surfaces).
Prevention: Care plans should address disease-specific preventive measures and risk factors for pressure injuries, including sensory perception, shear, moisture, nutrition, and patient mobility.
Preference: Preference considers the preferences of the patient and the patient's caregivers. For example, the patient may choose a "position of comfort" resulting in greater potential for skin breakdown.
Adapted from SCALE: Skin Changes at Life's End[1]

References
1. Sibbald RG, Krasner DL, Lutz J. SCALE: Skin changes at life's end: final consensus statement: October 1, 2009. *Adv Skin Wound Care.* 2010;23(5):225-236.
2. Reuben DB, Tinetti ME. Goal-oriented patient care – an alternative health outcomes paradigm. *N Engl J Med.* 2012;366:777-779.
3. Krasner DL, Rodeheaver GT, Sibbald RG. Interprofessional wound caring. In Krasner DL, Rodeheaver GT, Sibbald RG, eds. *Chronic Wound Care: A Clinical Sourcebook for Healthcare Professionals.* 4th ed. Malvern, PA: HMP Communications; 2007:3-9.

COMMUNICATION

Communication is critical when identifying goals of care. The BUILD™ Model provides a framework for communication to create a dialogue between clinician, patient, and caregiver. This communication model assists in initiating and facilitating a difficult conversation by gaining patient trust and respect. Ultimately, the discussion that ensues allows clinician, patient, and caregiver to BUILD™ the goals of care.[1] The following table provides sample conversation starters and talking points using the BUILD Model.

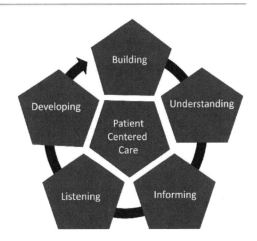

Figure 2. The BUILD Model

Developing Goals of Care Using the BUILD Model[1]		
Component	**Description**	**Key Conversation Points & Phrases**
BUILD the foundation	Build trust and respect	• "Thank you for talking with me today" • "I appreciate you sharing your thoughts with me" • "This must be very difficult for you" • "Are you ready to talk about this?"
UNDERSTAND the patient	Understand how the wound impacts the patient and family	• "What are you hoping hospice can do for you?" • "Help me understand what you'd like to see happen" • "I want to make sure we're on the same page" • "How can I be of help today?" • "Tell me what you understand about your wound right now"
INFORM the patient	Provide information on wound treatment and expected outcomes	• Wound treatment risks and benefits • Disease progression • Role of the hospice team members
LISTEN to the patient	Listen as the patient shares wound care goals; use active listening techniques	• "How is this wound impacting your quality of life?" • "How is wound care impacting your quality of life?" • "Tell me what you are noticing about your wound" • "What wound treatments have or have not been helpful?"
DEVELOP a plan with the patient	Develop a plan of care including the patient, family, hospice, and patient's circle of caregivers	• Negotiate treatment plan • "This is a process, not an event" • Acknowledge the patient/family as decision-makers • Agree to disagree • Revisit the topic on an ongoing basis

Reference

1. Collier KS, Kimbrel JM, Protus BM. Medication appropriateness at end-of-life: a new tool for balancing medicine and communication for optimal outcomes: the BUILD model. *Home Healthc Nurse*. 2013;31(9):518-524.

EDUCATION

A critical step in initiating any plan of care is education. Patient education begins with assessment of the patient's knowledge base and then BUILDing on this foundation. Just as BUILDing the goals of care are patient-centered, education must also be patient-centered. Printed materials are time-savers; however, when developing them, carefully consider the patient and caregiver's education level, health literacy, culture, and language.[1] BUILD on the patient and caregiver's current knowledge of the wound and its care.

At the end of life, education should focus on the emotional and psychological impact the wound has on the patient and family. Wound pain, odor, and exudate have the potential to cause significant social isolation and embarrassment for both the patient and the family. Often, wound care falls to a single caregiver, which may result in that caregiver feeling isolated. If the wound deteriorates, the caregiver may be criticized by other family members even though the deterioration is related to disease process rather than inadequate care. Patients are often embarrassed by the odor, leakage of fluid from the wound, and the unpleasant appearance of the wound. Consciously or subconsciously, wounds are often perceived as a failure on the part of patient or caregiver to provide adequate care or as a betrayal of one's own body. The wound is a constant reminder of the presence of disease and the dis-ease it creates. Providing education to the patient and the patient's circle of care will help reduce or eliminate these concerns. This circle of care includes family members, caregivers in the home, or facility staff (e.g., extended care facilities or assisted living facilities).

All members of the hospice interdisciplinary team may facilitate communication, assist in collaboration, and provide education in managing the patient's skin care needs. Critical components of patient education include:[2]

- Identifying barriers to learning, including cultural, physical, emotional, or environmental obstacles
- Defining the learning style of patient and caregivers; use this learning style to provide education
- Determining the patient's ability to read and understand the presented material
- Identifying the learning needs of the patient, including current knowledge level and beliefs
- Identifying the patient and caregiver's readiness to learn
- Defining the learning goals of the patient and caregiver
- Managing physical symptoms that may impede learning, such as pain or dyspnea
- Reinforcing education at every visit

Clinician education is also necessary. Lack of knowledge is one of the most common barriers associated with a failed plan of care. Also, pressure injury incidence increases if clinician knowledge is insufficient. Clinician training should be repeated at regular intervals to address both staff changes and guideline modifications.[3] The clinician must assume responsibility for self-education and recognize it is not a one-time event. Best education practices also help patients and families formulate realistic expectations about their wound treatments, risks, and healing.

References

1. Nix DP, Peirce B. Noncompliance, nonadherence, or barriers to a sustainable plan? In Bryant RA, Nix DP, eds. *Acute & Chronic Wounds: Current Management Concepts.* 4th ed. St Louis, MO:Elsevier/Mosby; 2012:408-415.
2. Thomas Hess C. *Clinical Guide to Skin & Wound Care.* 7th ed. Ambler, PA: Lippincott Williams & Wilkins; 2013.
3. Ayello EA, Capitulo KL, Fowler E, et al. Legal issues in the care of pressure ulcer patients: key concepts for health care providers: a consensus paper from the International Expert Wound Care Advisory Panel. *J Palliat Med.* 2009;12(11):995-1008.

ASSESSMENT AND DOCUMENTATION

GOALS

- Describe the fundamental components of skin and wound assessments
- Demonstrate complete documentation of skin and wound assessments
- Discuss the key issues surrounding wound photography

DEFINITIONS

Assessment refers to the process of evaluating the characteristics and qualities of a person. Assessment provides the essential information regarding a patient and their health status, and serves as the foundation for developing a plan of care. Perform initial and ongoing skin and wound assessments for all patients at regular intervals and with any change in condition.[1] Document assessment findings to reflect standards of care and aid in communication between members of the interdisciplinary group. Standardize skin and wound assessment documentation to capture all areas of the assessment and develop an individualized plan of care for each patient.[2]

SKIN AND WOUND ASSESSMENT

Conduct and document skin and wound assessments upon admission, at regular intervals, and with any change in patient condition. In the extended care setting, facility staff may perform a skin assessment daily, while in homecare and hospice, skin assessment usually occurs with each nursing visit. Perform wound assessments weekly and with any change in patient condition. Regulatory agencies and organizational policies dictate assessment frequency. Specifically, The Centers for Medicare & Medicaid Services (CMS) Hospice Conditions of Participation mandates completion of a comprehensive patient assessment upon admission and, at a minimum, every 15 days thereafter.[3] This should include a skin and wound assessment. In the long-term care setting, CMS recommends documentation of wounds, at minimum, weekly.[4] Organizational policies may be more stringent in assessment frequency. Monitoring occurs daily and indicates a change in condition that warrants more frequent assessment and documentation, as well as documentation of physician and patient/family notification, and any subsequent changes in wound care orders.[1]

Conduct a skin assessment by inspecting and palpating the skin to evaluate for changes in temperature, color, moisture, turgor, or texture. Pay close attention to areas prone to friction, moisture, and pressure, including areas of skin near medical devices, such as urinary catheters, feeding tubes, and oxygen delivery devices. Document the presence of bruising, lesions, pruritic areas, edema, traumatic injuries, or pain. Because all areas of the skin must be assessed, coordinate the skin assessment with daily grooming and hygiene.[1]

Document any extrinsic or intrinsic factors contributing to or as a potential cause of skin breakdown. Extrinsic factors contributing to skin breakdown include environmental concerns, such as a poorly fitted wheelchair, inappropriate mattress, or problematic devices, such as splints or braces. Intrinsic factors contributing to skin breakdown include the patient's mobility status, disease prognosis, continence status, or nutritional status, to name just a few. A risk assessment tool identifies risk factors for skin breakdown, specifically, pressure injuries.[1] See *Resource List*, page 119 for a list of risk assessment tools.

After conducting a comprehensive skin assessment, perform a wound assessment. The required components of a wound assessment include a description of the wound bed, wound edge, and periwound tissue as well as an evaluation of the holistic patient *(see table on page 7)*. Begin a comprehensive wound assessment by characterizing the wound bed. Define the etiology, the location, the chronicity, the size, the tissue, the amount of exudate, and any signs or symptoms of infection, odor, or pain present in the wound bed. Then move to the wound edge and assess for undermining, tunneling, epibole, or maceration. Moving outward from the wound bed and wound edge, evaluate the surrounding tissue and note if it is intact, denuded, edematous, firm, indurated, pale, or reddened. Finally, evaluate the holistic patient,

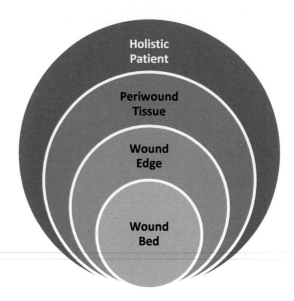

Figure 1. Components of Wound Assessment

noting any preventive measures, comorbidities, goals of care, educational needs, and outcomes of the current interventions. [1,2,5,6]

Note that wound healing is traditionally the desired outcome of wound care, and the wound assessment provides indicators of wound healing; however, for the palliative care patient, the wound may or may not heal. The likelihood of the wound healing is determined using the F.R.A.I.L. Healing Probability Assessment Tool.[7] The more risk factors present, the less likely the wound will heal. Educating the patient and family on the results of this tool allows for the creation of realistic wound care goals that focus on symptom relief while allowing the patient to enjoy a higher quality of life.[7] Identifying the healing probability also serves as the foundation for creating realistic goals of care, whether they be prescription, preservation, palliation, prevention, or patient preference.[5]

Components of a Comprehensive Wound Assessment[1,2,5-7]	
Assessment Area	**Specific Documentation**

Wound Bed	**Wound Type, Age, and Location**
	• Pressure injury, lower extremity ulcer (venous, arterial, neuropathic), traumatic wound (skin tear, laceration), malignant wound; superficial, partial thickness, or full thickness
	• Acute versus chronic wound
	• Use correct anatomical location (e.g., right lateral malleolus)
	Wound Size
	• Document Length x Width x Depth in centimeters
	   ○ Length: measure head to toe
	   ○ Width: measure side to side
	   ○ Depth: measure deepest depth (only if the wound bed is visible)
	Wound Bed Tissue
	• Use: slough (devitalized tissue, yellow/brown/grey), eschar (necrotic tissue, black), granulation tissue (red, healthy tissue), epithelial tissue (pale pink, epithelial cells)
	• Describe in percentages (e.g., 40% slough and 60% granulation tissue)
	Exudate Type
	• Serous: thin, watery exudate
	• Serosanguineous: thin, red exudate
	• Sanguineous: bloody exudate
	• Purulent: pus-like exudate
	Exudate Amount
	• None: dry wound bed
	• Scant: wound is moist but no exudate is present on dressing
	• Light/Small: wound bed is moist and < 25% of the dressing has exudate present
	• Moderate: wound bed is wet and 25 - 75% of the dressing has exudate present
	• Heavy/Copious: wound bed is wet and ≥ 75% of the dressing has exudate present
	Odor
	• Describe odor: foul, pungent, absent, strong, sweet
	Signs/Symptoms of Infection *(see page 19)*
	• Superficial (NERDS) versus deeper or possible systemic (STONES)
	Pain
	• Document current pain assessment and nonpharmacological and pharmacological interventions. See treatment grids for additional management recommendations. Base interventions on type of pain:
	   ○ Noncyclic acute (associated with a one-time procedure), cyclic acute (associated with recurring procedures), or chronic wound pain (may be nociceptive or neuropathic)

Wound Edge	**Tunneling/Undermining** • Measure depth in centimeters, describe location using clock system: head 12 o'clock, toes 6 o'clock **Defining Characteristics** • Defined/undefined, attached/detached, rolled (epibole), dry, macerated, shape (regular, irregular)
Periwound Tissue	• Describe the appearance of surrounding tissue: intact, denuded, edematous, firm, indurated, pale, reddened

Holistic Patient	• **Preventive Measures:** describe preventive measures currently in place: dietary modifications, support surface, turning/repositioning schedule, heel suspension, incontinence care, barrier creams, laboratory monitoring
	• **Comorbidities/Contributing Factors:** patient prognosis or preference, diagnoses, limitations to repositioning/offloading pressure, nutritional status, infection, mobility status, medications
	• **Goals of Care:** prescription, preservation, palliation, prevention, patient preference
	• **Outcome of Care:**
	   ○ Consider if orders are appropriate for present wound condition and are improving quality of life
	   ○ Document evidence of healing or deterioration – Pressure Ulcer Scale for Healing (PUSH©) displays healing graphically for pressure injuries if healing is a goal of care.[8]
	   ○ Document impact on quality of life and any interventions to improve symptoms
	   ○ Document notification of physician/patient/responsible party and any new orders received
	• **Education:** document the education provided to patient

DOCUMENTATION

Document skin and wound assessments in the patient's medical record using consistent descriptions of the wound characteristics, including exudate and odor. Timely documentation of skin and wound assessments allows for continuity of care. Consistent and accurate documentation of skin and wound assessments provides support to the appropriateness of continuing the current plan of care or the need to change the plan of care.[1] The following is an example of narrative documentation of a pressure injury:

> *Stage 3 pressure injury to the sacrum measuring 2.4 x 3.5 x 0.4 cm. Wound bed with 60% granulation tissue and 40% slough. Moderate serous drainage. No odor noted. Wound edges attached but macerated from 3 o'clock to 10 o'clock. No epibole, undermining, or tunneling. Surrounding tissue is warm, dry, and intact. PAINAD pain score 1/10 during wound assessment. Current preventive measures include turning and repositioning frequently (family attempts to turn every 2 to 4 hours), floating heels while in bed, and use of a pressure-redistributing support surface. The patient is incontinent of urine and stool. Incontinence care is provided with each incontinent episode. Barrier cream is applied twice daily and PRN incontinence. Comorbidities include anemia and hypertension. The patient is ordered comfort medications only. The patient eats approximately 25% of all pureed meals, is fed by family, and drinks sips of nectar-thickened liquid throughout the day. Weight is stable at 114 pounds. The patient is bed bound. FAST score is a 7f and PPS is 20%. Family wishes to maintain patient's comfort and state that the most distressing symptom is exudate. Current treatment order is amorphous hydrogel daily. Physician notified of current wound assessment and order received to cleanse pressure injury to sacrum with normal saline solution, pat periwound tissue dry, apply liquid barrier film to periwound tissue, loosely pack dead space of wound with calcium alginate, secure with bordered foam dressing, change every three days and as needed if soiled. Family notified of new orders, education provided on the application of the treatment, return demonstration acceptable. The patient tolerated wound assessment and dressing application well.*

WOUND PHOTOGRAPHY

Wound photography serves as an adjunct to wound assessment and diagnosis or as a method to minimize legal liability in a variety of healthcare settings.[9] Although used to reduce legal liability, states vary on their stance regarding the use of photographs in court. Therefore, wound imaging should not replace the need for accurate written documentation. The Wound Ostomy and Continence Nurses Society® recommends the use of photography only to augment current written documentation of the wound. This organization has developed the Photography in Wound Documentation: Fact Sheet that addresses issues, such as informed consent, guidelines for the use of cell phones as an imaging device, and confidentiality. Referencing this information sheet is imperative before instituting wound photography in an organization.[10]

KEY POINTS

- Inspect and palpate the skin regularly to evaluate for changes in temperature, color, moisture, turgor, or texture, or the presence of bruising, lesions, pruritic areas, edema, traumatic injuries, or pain.
- Comprehensive wound assessment includes the characteristics of the wound, holistic patient assessment, an estimate of the wound's ability to heal, and impact on the patient's quality of life.
- Document skin and wound assessments in a timely manner to allow for continuity of care among the members of the interdisciplinary group.
- Wound photography does not replace the need for accurate written skin and wound documentation.

References

1. Nix DP. Skin and wound inspection and assessment. In Bryant RA, Nix DP, eds. *Acute & Chronic Wounds: Current Management Concepts.* 4th ed. St Louis, MO:Elsevier/Mosby; 2012:108-121.
2. Keast DH, Bowering K, Evans AW, et al. MEASURE: a proposed assessment framework for developing best practice recommendations for wound assessment. *Wound Repair Regen.* 2004;12(3):S1-S17.
3. Centers for Medicare & Medicaid Services (CMS). Medicare and Medicaid Programs: Hospice Conditions of Participation; Final Rule. Initial and comprehensive assessment of the patient. *Fed Regist* 2008;73(109):32101-32110. Codified at 42 CFR 418.54.
4. Centers for Medicare & Medicaid Services (CMS). State Operators Manual. Appendix PP - Guidance to Surveyors for Long Term Care Facilities. Pub. 100-07 (Rev. 168, 03-08-17); 266. Available at: https://www.cms.gov/Regulations-and-Guidance/Guidance/Manuals/downloads/som107ap_pp_guidelines_ltcf.pdf Accessed October 19, 2017.
5. Sibbald RG, Krasner DL, Lutz J. SCALE: Skin changes at life's end: final consensus statement: October 1, 2009. *Adv Skin Wound Care.* 2010;23(5):225-236.
6. National Pressure Ulcer Advisory Panel (NPUAP), European Pressure Ulcer Advisory Panel (EPUAP) and Pan Pacific Pressure Injury Alliance. Prevention and Treatment of Pressure Ulcers: Quick Reference Guide. Emily Haesler (Ed.). Cambridge Media: Osborne Park, Western Australia; 2014.
7. F.R.A.I.L. [Internet] Palliative Wound Care and Healing Probability Assessment Tool. Available at: http://www.frailcare.org/images/Palliative%20Wound%20Care.pdf Accessed May 12, 2017.
8. National Pressure Ulcer Advisory Panel (NPUAP). PUSH Tool 3.0 (web version). Available at: http://www.npuap.org/resources/educational-and-clinical-resources/push-tool/push-tool/ Accessed April 9, 2018
9. Brown G. Wound documentation: managing risk. *Adv Skin Wound Care.* 2006;19(3):155-165.
10. Wound Ostomy and Continence Nurses Society (WOCN). Photography in wound documentation: fact sheet. [Internet].http://c.ymcdn.com/sites/www.wocn.org/resource/resmgr/Publications/Photography_in_Wound_Documen.pdf. Accessed May 12, 2017.

ANATOMY AND PHYSIOLOGY OF SKIN

GOALS

- Identify major components of skin that play a role in maintaining physiological equilibrium
- Describe the structure and function of each layer of skin

DEFINITIONS

Skin is the largest organ of the body and, as such, serves to protect an individual from the environment while maintaining physiological equilibrium. Because of the critical role skin plays in maintaining homeostasis, any compromise to skin integrity can be life-threatening and debilitating. Characteristics of skin will vary depending upon the unique attributes of an individual, such as the pigment of their skin or the current disease state. Additionally, the thickness of skin will vary depending upon anatomical location. Understanding the anatomy and physiology of the skin is essential to competently assessing and documenting wounds, staging pressure injuries, and distinguishing partial thickness from full thickness wounds.[1,2]

ANATOMY AND PHYSIOLOGY

The epidermis is the visible external layer of the skin. It is comprised of five layers. The innermost layer, the stratum basale, is one cell layer thick. The cells of the stratum basale undergo mitosis to form keratinocytes and slowly migrate to the skin surface while undergoing transformation through each layer of the epidermis. Above the stratum basale are the stratum spinosum, stratum granulosum, and stratum lucidum (only present in some areas). These three layers contain keratinocytes in progressive stages of differentiation and flattening as they migrate towards the skin surface. The end product of this differentiation process is the stratum corneum, which consists of dead, flattened, waterproof cells called corneocytes. The creation of the stratum corneum allows the epidermis to serve as an impermeable barrier to the external world – both keeping water in and from preventing the entry of water, microorganisms, and chemicals.[1]

The basement membrane, located between the epidermis and dermis, is comprised of two layers, the lamina lucida and lamina densa. The basement membrane serves as a junction between the epidermis and dermis to decrease the potential for shearing injury. The junction also serves as a barrier; however, cells involved in the inflammatory process, cancerous cells, and some bacteria can travel through the basement membrane.[1]

The dermis is the next layer of skin. The dermis consists of two layers – the papillary layer and the reticular layer. The papillary layer is thin and contains collagen fibers, fine elastic fibers, and ground substance. The reticular layer is thick and contains collagen bundles and coarse elastic fibers. The presence of collagen and elastin throughout the dermis provides the skin with strength and elasticity. The ground substance serves as a medium for the three primary cells found in the dermis – fibroblasts, histiocytes, and mast cells. The fibroblast is the fundamental cell of the dermis and produces collagen, elastin, and ground substance. Fibroblasts also play a role in the wound healing cascade. Histiocytes remove debris created as a result of the inflammatory process. Mast cells are a type of white blood cell involved in immune response and wound healing.[1]

Below the dermis lies subcutaneous tissue. The subcutaneous tissue serves as an area for fat storage with the presence of adipocytes separated by connective tissue. It also contains nerves, blood vessels, and lymphatic vessels. The fat stored in the subcutaneous tissue serves as a source of energy for the body, pads and protects the body from injury, and insulates the body from the cold.[1]

KEY POINTS

- Skin is the largest organ of the body and serves to maintain homeostasis.
- The epidermis serves as a waterproof barrier and, when intact, prevents the passage of bacteria and chemicals.
- The basement membrane anchors the epidermis to the dermis.
- The dermis is comprised of the papillary and reticular layer, which contain collagen and provide strength and elasticity to the skin.
- The subcutaneous tissue serves as an area for fat storage, which provides energy, protects from injury, and insulates the body from the cold.

References

1. Fang RC, Mustoe TA. Structure and function of the skin. In: Guyuron B, Eriksson E, Persing JA, Chung KC, Disa JJ, Gosain AK, Kinney BM, Rubin JP. *Plastic Surgery: Indications and Practice*. Philadelphia, PA:Saunders/Elsevier;2009: 105-112.
2. Bryant RA, Nix DP, eds. *Acute & Chronic Wounds: Current Management Concepts.* 4th ed. St Louis, MO:Elsevier/Mosby; 2012.

PHASES OF WOUND HEALING

GOALS

- Describe the concepts that serve as the framework for wound healing
- Describe the phases of wound healing
- Identify factors that lead to chronic wounds

DEFINITIONS

Wound healing is a complicated process that is not fully understood; however, the understanding of wound healing has increased significantly over the past few decades, providing knowledge regarding the concepts of regeneration versus scar formation, partial thickness versus full thickness wounds, acute versus chronic wounds, and healing by various intentions.[1]

Regeneration versus Scar Formation
Fundamental to the understanding of wound healing are the concepts of regeneration and scar formation. **Regeneration** refers to the process of replacing lost tissue with a replica. **Scar formation** refers to the method of repairing lost tissue with connective tissue that forms a scar over the wound bed. Because the skin's ability to heal by regeneration is limited, most wounds heal by scar formation. These concepts are central to the understanding that pressure injuries do not heal by reverse staging.[1]

Partial Thickness versus Full Thickness Wounds
Partial thickness wounds affect only the epidermis and the superficial layers of the dermis. **Full thickness** wounds affect all layers of the skin and extend into the subcutaneous tissue, muscle, or bone. The healing process and the time required to heal will differ depending on if the wound is full or partial thickness.[1]

Acute versus Chronic Wounds
Acute wounds heal without complication, usually within four weeks. They may originate from trauma or surgery. A skin tear is one example of an acute wound. On the other hand, **chronic wounds** fail to progress through the healing cascade in an orderly fashion. Healing stalls in one phase of the process, such as the inflammatory phase, and usually takes longer than four weeks.[1]

Healing by Primary versus Secondary Intention
There are multiple types of wound healing. In palliative care, wounds usually heal by secondary intention, and occasionally primary intention may be used. Wound healing by **primary intention** refers to the process of healing where wound edges are close to one another allowing the epithelial cells to migrate from the wound edges and rapidly close the wound. This process is fast and may be complete in as little as three days. This type of healing is beneficial because it reduces the risk of developing an infection and minimizes the formation of scar tissue. An example of a wound healing by primary intention is a laceration that is closed by sutures.[1] Wound healing by **secondary intention** refers to the process of healing when the wound edges are open. The defect is gradually filled in with scar tissue. Healing by secondary intention results in greater scar tissue formation, and, because of the time required to heal, these wounds are at greater risk of developing an infection.[1]

WOUND HEALING PHASES

Normal healing of a full thickness, acute wound involves a progression through four distinct phases: hemostasis, inflammation, proliferation, and remodeling. Although described in separate stages, in actuality, these stages may overlap with one another.[2,3] Due to intrinsic or extrinsic factors, a wound may fail to progress in an orderly fashion through these four stages resulting in a chronic wound.[2] A review of the four phases is warranted to understand wound healing and the complications that can arise during the wound healing process resulting in a chronic wound.

Hemostasis, the first phase of wound healing, occurs immediately after tissue injury. Simply defined, the process of hemostasis begins when platelets from damaged blood vessels undergo activation and aggregate together to form a clot to control bleeding. Removal of the clot occurs after vessel wall repair is complete. Cytokines are then secreted to initiate the inflammatory phase of wound healing.[3-5]

The **inflammatory** phase usually begins between one to four days after injury. Vasodilation allows neutrophils to move into the wound with the primary purpose of removing bacteria and debris from the wound bed.[3] This vasodilation can cause wounds to become red and swollen or warm and tender, which may be mistaken for an infection.[6] Macrophages eventually replace neutrophils and continue to clean bacteria and debris from the wound bed. After achieving a clean wound bed, macrophages secrete cytokines and growth factors that signal the transition from the inflammatory phase to the proliferative phase.[3]

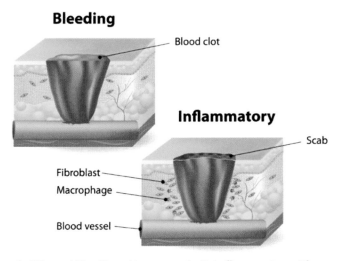

Figure 1. Wound Healing: Hemostasis & Inflammatory Phases

The **proliferative** phase can last from four to 21 days post-injury. During this phase, macrophages and other cells secrete growth factors that signal fibroblasts to migrate to the area. The fibroblasts begin production of collagen and proteoglycans, which ultimately results in the development of granulation tissue filling the wound bed. The growth of capillaries supports the new granulation tissue.[4] To bring the wound edges closer together, a unique process called **contraction** occurs. Fibroblasts are responsible for contraction by differentiating into myofibroblasts. The myofibroblasts possess characteristics of smooth muscle, which allows them to contract and bring the wound edges closer together.[4] Epithelial cells are stimulated to move across the wound bed from the wound edges through the loss of cellular contact. Epithelial cells will begin to migrate across a wound bed in as little as a few hours after the initial injury. Contact with other epithelial cells, referred to as **contact inhibition**, signals the epithelial cells to stop migrating.[6]

Note that this re-epithelialization process relates to epithelialization in **full thickness** wounds or wounds that extend beyond the dermis and possibly go as deep as muscle or bone. In contrast, **partial thickness** wounds, defined as a wound that may extend down into but not through the dermis, will have the possibility of epithelialization occurring not only at the wound margins but also at skin appendages, which are lined with epidermal cells, resulting in islands of epithelial tissue throughout the wound bed.[4]

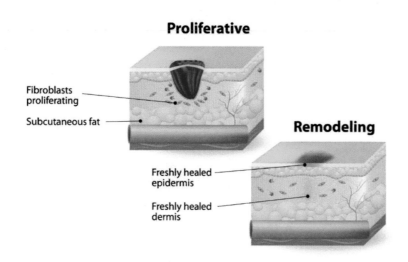

Proliferative

Fibroblasts proliferating

Subcutaneous fat

Remodeling

Freshly healed epidermis

Freshly healed dermis

Figure 2. Wound Healing: Proliferative & Remodeling Phases

The final stage of the wound healing process is **remodeling**. Once disorganized, collagen fibers are now organized to increase the strength of the scar tissue. This process may continue for several years after the initial injury. An important point to remember in the process of healing is that the body does not replace the lost layers of skin with a replica. Instead, scar tissue is formed, which consists of densely packed collagen fibers. This scar tissue increases in tensile strength throughout the remodeling process but will never have the strength of the original skin before the injury. Typically, this scar tissue will have just 80% of the strength of undamaged skin.[2]

CAUSES OF CHRONIC WOUNDS

Realizing the complexity of the wound healing process, it is no surprise that some wounds fail to progress through these phases and become chronic. Historically, chronic wounds are thought to be trapped in the inflammatory stage. Multiple factors at the cellular level play a role in wounds being deemed chronic in nature. Some chronic wounds demonstrate a disruption in protease activity while others have an altered inflammatory response. They may also have fibroblasts with altered shapes, cells with decreased mitotic activity, or altered extracellular matrix, which prevents epithelialization.[2]

Additionally, disease states, age, medications, smoking, and inappropriate wound care practices play a role in delayed wound healing. For example, the edema associated with venous insufficiency results in ulcerations and often stalls wound healing. Advanced patient age results in a decrease in the percentage of replicating fibroblasts, and the fibroblasts that are present demonstrate impaired ability to produce extracellular matrix.[2] Medications, such as warfarin or steroids, impede wound healing by inhibiting one or more phases of the process (*see table page 15*). An individual's nutritional status, specifically weight loss and the presence of protein-calorie malnutrition, can stop the wound healing process completely.[7] Finally, inappropriate wound care practices, such as frequent or prolonged dressing changes, allow the wound bed to cool, delay healing, and increase a patient's risk of developing an infection.[8]

As a result of these changes, chronic wounds typically have wound beds with necrotic tissue, which invites bacteria to colonize the wound bed. If allowed to remain in the wound bed, the inflammatory response is prolonged and infection is possible, especially in patients with compromised immunity or who have diabetes. Additionally, bacteria can form a biofilm on the surface of the wound that prevents healing.[2]

Effects of Medication on Wound Healing[7,9,10]

IMPAIR: Medications That May Hinder Wound Healing			
Medication Class	**Examples**	**Mechanism**	**Comments**
Anti-inflammatory	Prednisone, hydrocortisone, dexamethasone, colchicine	Inhibits inflammatory phase of wound healing; impairs granulation and epithelial resurfacing	Corticosteroids help manage other symptoms (pain, appetite, etc.); evaluate risk vs. benefits with patient.
Immunosuppressant	Azathioprine, methotrexate, hydroxyurea	May inhibit inflammatory and proliferative phases of wound healing	May no longer be necessary at the end of life; evaluate risk vs. benefits with patient.
Antiseptics	Chlorhexidine, povidone iodine, hydrogen peroxide, acetic acid, Dakin's® solution	Change in pH; indiscriminate chemical destruction	Appropriate for cleansing but should not be left on wound bed; rinse with saline after cleansing to minimize toxic effects.
Antibiotics	Mupirocin, gentamicin, bacitracin, neomycin, polymyxin B	Topical antibiotics are bacteriostatic only	Topical antibiotics may cause allergic contact dermatitis. Potential for growth of resistant organisms
Cardiovascular -anticoagulants -vasoconstrictors	Warfarin, heparin, epinephrine, nicotine	Prevention of fibrin formation; Vasoconstrictors impair microcirculation	Anticoagulants: Wound healing delayed due to lack of fibrin formation. Vasoconstrictors: decrease blood supply to wound; may increase ulcer necrosis

ENHANCE: Medications That May Benefit Wound Healing			
Medication Class	**Examples**	**Mechanism**	**Comments**
Antiseptics	Chlorhexidine, povidone iodine, acetic acid, Dakin's® solution	Inhibit or destroy microorganisms	Chemical destructive agents to decontaminate wounds. Topical use only. Rinse wound bed with normal saline after use of antiseptics
Anti-epileptics	Phenytoin	Modifies collagen remodeling	May be compounded for topical wound application. See *Other Therapies*, page 111
Cardiovascular -antiplatelets -vasodilators	Aspirin, NSAIDs, calcium channel blockers	Enhance tissue perfusion through vasodilation or decreased platelet aggregation	Prevents tissue injury through inhibition of thrombus formation. Increases blood flow to ischemic tissue

KEY POINTS

- Most wounds heal by scar formation.
- Partial thickness wounds extend into the dermis while full thickness wounds extend through the dermis and into the subcutaneous tissue or deeper structures.
- The four phases of wound healing are hemostasis, inflammation, proliferation, and remodeling.
- Chronic wounds fail to progress through the phases of wound healing and usually become stuck in the inflammatory phase.
- Disease states, age, medications, nutrition, smoking, and inappropriate wound care practices can lead to the development of chronic wounds.

References

1. Bryant RA, Nix DP, eds. *Acute & Chronic Wounds: Current Management Concepts.* 4ᵗʰ ed. St Louis, MO:Elsevier/Mosby; 2012.
2. Enoch S, Price P. Cellular, molecular and biochemical differences in the pathophysiology of healing between acute wounds, chronic wounds and wounds in the aged. *World Wide Wounds.* August 2004. http://www.worldwidewounds.com/2004/august/Enoch/Pathophysiology-Of-Healing.html. Accessed April 12, 2017.
3. Nguyen DT, Orgill DP, Murphy GF. The pathophysiologic basis for wound healing and cutaneous regeneration. In: Orgill D, Blancos C, eds. *Biomaterials for Treating Skin Loss.* Cambridge, England: Woodhead; 2009:25-57.
4. Saxena V. Biomechanics of skin. In: Orgill D, Blancos C, eds. *Biomaterials for Treating Skin Loss.* Cambridge, England: Woodhead; 2009:18-24.
5. Versteeg HH, Heemskerk JWM, Levi M, et al. New fundamentals in hemostasis. *Phys Rev.* 2013;91(1):327-358.
6. Von Der Heyde RL, Evans RB. Wound classification and management. In: Skirven TM, Osterman AL, Fedorczyk JM, Amadio PC. *Rehabilitation of the Hand and Upper Extremity*. Philadelphia, PA: Mosby; 2011:219-232.
7. Levine JM. The effect of oral medication on wound healing. *Adv Skin Wound Care.* 2017;30(3):137-142.
8. Wound Care Education Institute (WCEI) Warm wound healing? It is all about foam dressings. [Internet]. http://blog.wcei.net/tag/moist-wound-dressing. Accessed May 15, 2017.
9. Karukonda SRK, Flynn TC, Boh EE, et al. The effects of drugs on wound healing- part II. Specific classes of drugs and their effect on healing wounds. *Int J Dermatol.* 2000;39:321-333.
10. Lexi-Drugs Online. Lexicomp. Wolters Kluwer; Hudson, OH. Accessed April 16, 2018

WOUND BED PREPARATION

GOALS

- Discuss the four components of wound bed preparation using the TIME mnemonic
- Identify methods of debridement and the indications and contraindications of each
- Identify the signs and symptoms of superficial and deeper wound infections and appropriate treatment modalities for each
- Discuss methods of adding, maintaining, and absorbing moisture in the wound bed
- Define characteristics of an unhealthy wound edge and appropriate wound care interventions

DEFINITIONS

Wound bed preparation refers to the systematic approach of addressing wound bed characteristics that cause the healing process to stall. The TIME mnemonic describes components of wound bed preparation:[1]

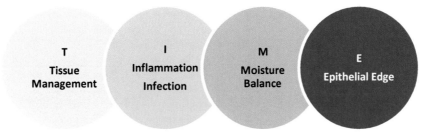

Figure 1. TIME Mnemonic for Wound Bed Preparation

Each component of wound bed preparation addresses a specific characteristic of the wound that impedes the wound healing process.[2] Although wound bed preparation has the ultimate goal of healing the wound, it is also beneficial to the palliative patient because it addresses aspects of wounds that may result in a reduced quality of life, such as pain, odor, and exudate. Therefore, discuss each component of wound bed preparation with the palliative patient to determine the treatment options that best meet their goals.

T – TISSUE MANAGEMENT (DEBRIDEMENT)

Tissue management, or debridement, refers to the removal of necrotic tissue and dead cells in the wound bed, such as slough and eschar.[5] Use one of five techniques to debride a wound – biosurgical, enzymatic, mechanical, autolytic, or sharp/surgical (*see table on page 18*).[5] Debride any wound, acute or chronic, when necrotic tissue or foreign bodies are present or when the wound is infected.[3,4] While debridement is a requirement for wound healing and often regarded as an intensive intervention, the patient's quality of life is also likely to be negatively impacted without debridement. The benefits of debridement for the patient at the end of life include less wound exudate and less frequent dressing changes, decreased wound odor, and reduced wound bioburden leading to a reduced risk of developing an infection. If necrotic tissue is present, the question should not be if debridement is appropriate but what type of debridement is necessary and in line with the patient's goals of care. Discontinue debridement when the wound bed is clean and viable tissue is present. General words of caution when considering a debridement method for the palliative care patient include:[1,5,9]

- Identify perfusion status before debriding any lower extremity wound (e.g., arterial ulcers).
- Do not debride dry, stable (non-infected) ischemic wounds, wounds with dry gangrene, or stable eschar (dry and firmly attached without exudate or fluctuance) especially when present on heels.

Summary of Current Debridement Methods

Method & Description	Indications	Cautious Use	Contraindications	Comments
Biosurgical[2,8] Larvae of *Lucilia sericata* secrete digestive juices containing proteolytic enzymes and collagenase to digest necrotic tissue	• Diabetic foot ulcers, ischemic leg ulcers, burns, osteomyelitis, pressure injuries, wet gangrene, and necrotizing fasciitis (after surgery)	• Dry wounds (may need to add moisture)	• Fistula present in wound; exposed arteries & veins; abdominal wounds near an organ; pyoderma gangrenosum; *Pseudomonas* infection	• Often contained within a net • Use gauze as secondary dressing • Leave on wound ≤ 3 days, change gauze daily
Enzymatic[6,7] Selectively digests collagen fibers of necrotic tissue, leaving granulation tissue unharmed; product: Santyl®	• Chronic wounds or extensive burns with any amount of necrotic tissue • Crosshatched eschar	• Untreated localized infection, wounds with persistent infection despite treatment • Dry wounds, heavily exudative wounds	• Sepsis • Concurrent use with some wound cleansers, dressings, and antibiotics	• Continue use until debridement is complete and granulation tissue is present – stop if no improvement in 10 to 14 days
Autolytic[5,9] Relies on the body's own mechanisms to breakdown necrotic tissue by creating a moist wound bed	• Uninfected wounds • Unknown tissue perfusion, ischemia • Anticoagulant use; bleeding potential • Terminally ill/palliative care because pain free	• Colonized or critically colonized wounds • Eschar or necrotic tissue covering more than 50% of the wound bed • Deep, cavitating wounds • Immunocompromise	• Deep wound infection or sepsis • Dry, stable eschar	• Exudate present: hydrocolloid, foam, NaCl-impregnated gauze, alginate, or gelling fiber dressing • No exudate: TenderWet Active®, hydrogel, transparent film
Mechanical[5,9] Non-selective physical removal of viable and non-viable tissue	• Uninfected to locally infected wounds • Necrotic tissue covering less than 50% of the wound bed	• Unknown tissue perfusion, ischemia • Extensive necrotic tissue or heavy exudate • Anticoagulant use; bleeding potential • Pain	• Sepsis, systemic infection; granulation or epithelial tissue covering wound bed; stable eschar	• Pulsed lavage, whirlpool therapy • Avoid wet-to-dry dressings • Debriding mitt
Surgical/Sharp[1,5,9] Removal of necrotic tissue using surgical instruments	• Infection – local or systemic • Need for rapid removal of necrotic tissue • Crosshatching eschar • Extensive necrotic tissue	• Unskilled clinician • Unknown tissue perfusion • Uncontrolled pain • Anticoagulant use • Immunocompromise	• Stable eschar, dry gangrene, ischemia • Uncontrolled bleeding potential • Inability to maintain a sterile field	• Scalpel, scissors • At bedside or in operating room

I – INFLAMMATION/INFECTION

Superficial versus Deeper Wound Infection

All wounds contain bacteria. Most bacteria enter the wound bed through environmental contamination, dressings, the patient's bodily fluids, or the hands of the patient or healthcare provider.[10] Identify wound infection by evaluating the level of bacterial burden, which is classified into four progressive categories – contamination, colonization, critical colonization, and infection. **Contamination** is the presence of inert bacteria in a wound. Bacteria are present, but they are not harming the host, and they are not replicating at this time. If these bacteria begin replicating without hurting the host, this is **colonization**.[1]

Critical colonization (increased bacterial burden), initiates the body's immune response (inflammation), which delays wound healing. Ideally, in a healable wound, the wound size should decrease 20-40% after four weeks of appropriate treatment and may heal in 12 weeks.[10] Increased exudate, bleeding, or odor is present. Tissue breakdown and gram-negative and anaerobic organisms produce a foul odor. Critical colonization indicates a local or superficial infection. Treat with antimicrobial dressings in addition to debridement, if in alignment with the goals and wishes of the patient. Note that the use of a topical antibiotic to treat wound infection is discouraged due to the potential for adverse reactions and antimicrobial resistance.[11]

Failure to halt the replication of bacteria seen in critical colonization will result in a deeper wound **infection**. Pain, erythema, edema, cellulitis, wound deterioration, increased exudate, or pus may be evident. If the infection continues to spread systemically, fever ensues.[1] With the presence of these symptoms, use topical agents and debridement to treat the infection; however, consider the addition of systemic antibiotics if it is in line with the patient's goals (*see Figure 2*) for antimicrobial classifications). The mnemonics NERDS and STONES may be helpful in the differentiation of superficially infected (critically colonized) versus deeper infections and impending sepsis:[10]

NERDS = superficial infection when 2-3 of below are present in the wound	
N	Non-healing
E	Exudate
R	Red and bleeding surface granulation tissue
D	Debris on surface (yellow or black necrotic tissue)
S	Smell – unpleasant odor from wound (differentiate from absorbent dressing odors)
Treatment: Topical antimicrobial dressings and debridement of necrotic tissue	
STONES = deeper wound infection when 2-3 of below are present in the wound	
S	Size of wound is bigger
T	Temperature is elevated
O	"O's" Probe to exposed bone, or "Os" – Latin root for opening, or "Osteo" – Latin root for bone
N	New areas of breakdown
E	Exudate, erythema, edema
S	Smell
Treatment: Systemic antibiotics with topical antimicrobial dressings and debridement of necrotic tissue	

Adapted with permission from Sibbald et al[10]

If an infection requires the use of a systemic antibiotic, the results of a swab culture assist in selecting the appropriate antibiotic. The Levine method is the preferred technique for obtaining a swab culture. To perform the Levine method, apply gentle pressure to the wound bed using a culture swab while rotating the swab over a one centimeter square area of the wound bed (not the necrotic tissue).[10]

Host resistance often determines if an infection will occur. Host resistance is the ability of the host to resist bacterial invasion and damage by mounting an immune response. Systemic and local factors decrease host resistance. Systemically, an inadequate blood supply (blood perfusion to the wound), uncontrolled edema, vascular insufficiency, poorly controlled diabetes, smoking, poor nutrition, excess alcohol intake, immunodeficiency disease, and drugs that interfere with the immune system (*see table page 15*) decrease host resistance.[9] At the site of the wound, factors that contribute to infection and impair wound healing include the presence of foreign bodies, large wound size, and untreated, deeper infections, such as osteomyelitis. Patients at the end of life may have little ability to resist infection, and the presence of infection can result in distressing symptoms that reduce their quality of life. Additionally, infection poses a threat to life, especially in this vulnerable population.[9] Therefore, use best practices for the treatment and prevention of infections if these are in line with the patient's wishes, including:[10,12]

- Using wound culture or tissue biopsy to determine appropriate systemic antibiotic. Bacterial growth of 10^6 results in delayed wound healing. Wound culture is not used to diagnose infection.
- Determining level of bacterial burden (superficial infection, infection in the deep wound bed, or systemic infection – use NERDS and STONES).
- Using topical antimicrobial dressings and debridement for superficial infection (NERDS). Monitor response to treatment.
- Using systemic agents plus topical antimicrobial dressings and debridement for deep infection (STONES). Monitor response to treatment.
- Limiting antibacterial agent use to no longer than 14 days without weighing the benefits and risks of their use.
- Using good handwashing practices with every patient contact.

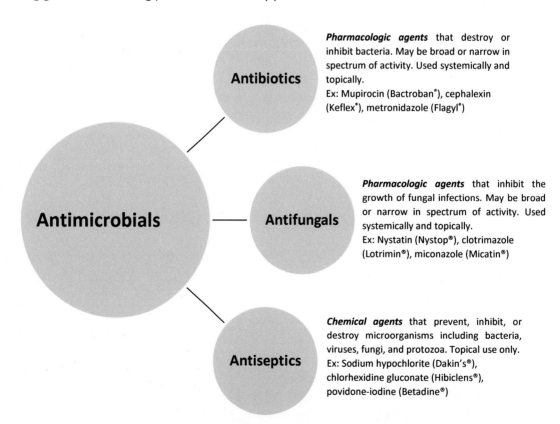

Antibiotics

Pharmacologic agents that destroy or inhibit bacteria. May be broad or narrow in spectrum of activity. Used systemically and topically.
Ex: Mupirocin (Bactroban®), cephalexin (Keflex®), metronidazole (Flagyl®)

Antimicrobials

Antifungals

Pharmacologic agents that inhibit the growth of fungal infections. May be broad or narrow in spectrum of activity. Used systemically and topically.
Ex: Nystatin (Nystop®), clotrimazole (Lotrimin®), miconazole (Micatin®)

Antiseptics

Chemical agents that prevent, inhibit, or destroy microorganisms including bacteria, viruses, fungi, and protozoa. Topical use only.
Ex: Sodium hypochlorite (Dakin's®), chlorhexidine gluconate (Hibiclens®), povidone-iodine (Betadine®)

Figure 2. Antimicrobial Classifications: Comparison of Antibiotic, Antifungal, and Antiseptic Activity

Biofilms

Biofilms may be the culprit when a superficial infection (critical colonization) is suspected. They represent colonies of various bacteria and other organisms living within a protective matrix attached to the wound surface. The body responds to the presence of a biofilm by initiating an inflammatory reaction; however, this inflammatory response is unable to affect the bacteria living within the protective matrix. Additionally, antibiotics, some topical wound care products, and antiseptics (sodium hypochlorite, acetic acid, alcohol, or hydrogen peroxide) cannot destroy the biofilm; as a result, wound healing stalls or deteriorates. Biofilm can be invisible to the naked eye or become large enough that it will appear as a thin, slimy layer present on the wound surface. Suspect a biofilm in all chronic, non-healing wounds.[13, 14]

Unfortunately, the concept of biofilms is relatively new, and the best method of treating biofilms is unknown. The current research supports frequent debridement as the best method of disrupting the biofilm. The debridement process disrupts the protective membrane of the organisms and represents a window of opportunity to intervene with topical antimicrobial dressings. A single method of debridement will usually not be successful in removing the biofilm, and the biofilm is capable of reforming within hours and maturing within a few days. Therefore, debridement needs to occur frequently, although the exact frequency has yet to be defined.[13,14]

Historically, sharp debridement is used to disrupt the biofilm followed by the application of an antimicrobial dressing to prevent reformation; however, as research continues, additional methods of disrupting biofilms are evolving, including the use of topical wound care products, solutions, and surfactants.[13,14] Additional methods of disrupting a biofilm currently being explored include:

- Irrigating and soaking the wound with a betaine and polyhexanide (PHMB) surfactant (Prontosan®) or hypochlorous acid solution (Vashe® Wound Therapy Solution)[13,15-17] followed by the application of an antimicrobial dressing.
- Betaine and polyhexanide (PHMB) gel (Prontosan® gel) applied as primary dressing daily.[13,15]
- Impregnating a primary dressing with hypochlorous acid solution (Vashe® Wound Therapy Solution) and changing the dressing daily.[16,17]
- Using a debriding mitt to mechanically debride the wound instead of sharp debridement.[18]
- Applying cadexomer iodine (Iodosorb® – effective against *Pseudomonas aeruginosa*).[19]

M – MOISTURE BALANCE

A moist wound bed is imperative to wound healing. A wound bed that is too dry results in cell death and slows epithelialization. A wound bed that is too wet macerates the periwound tissue and contains proteases that lengthen the inflammatory phase and slow wound healing. For the palliative patient, management of wound exudate also improves quality of life. Poor exudate management results in frequent dressing changes, and a dry wound bed is painful.[5] Therefore, selecting the correct product to manage exudate is not only a part of healing the wound but is imperative to managing distressing symptoms faced at the end of life. Topical wound care products offer a range of absorptive capacities. Select a product that manages the current exudate level while minimizing the number of dressing changes required. See Figure 3 to assist in choosing the correct product based on the level of exudate.

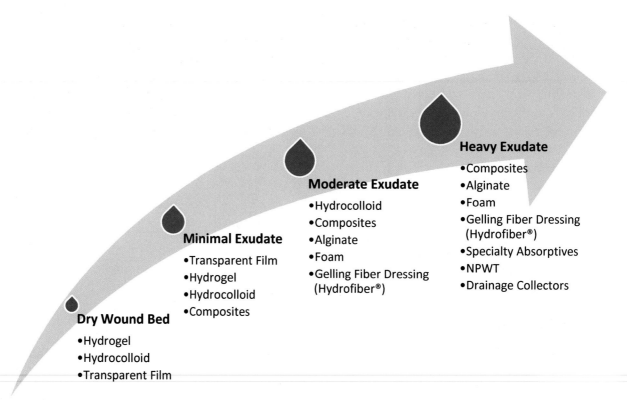

Heavy Exudate
- Composites
- Alginate
- Foam
- Gelling Fiber Dressing (Hydrofiber®)
- Specialty Absorptives
- NPWT
- Drainage Collectors

Moderate Exudate
- Hydrocolloid
- Composites
- Alginate
- Foam
- Gelling Fiber Dressing (Hydrofiber®)

Minimal Exudate
- Transparent Film
- Hydrogel
- Hydrocolloid
- Composites

Dry Wound Bed
- Hydrogel
- Hydrocolloid
- Transparent Film

Figure 3. Dressing Selection by Level of Exudate

In addition to exudate level, exudate viscosity should play a role in wound product selection. Exudate can range in thickness from thin and watery (low viscosity) to thick and sticky (high viscosity). High viscosity exudate is indicative of high protein content, usually due to bacterial infection or initiation of the inflammatory response. Treatment of the infection with a topical antimicrobial dressing and/or systemic antibiotic would serve to reduce the viscosity and volume of exudate. If, however, the high viscosity of exudate is due to sloughing of necrotic tissue, management of the exudate would concentrate on debridement.[20]

E – EPITHELIAL EDGE

Epithelial edge refers to factors that reduce the ability of the epithelial margin to migrate across the wound bed. Epithelial migration requires the wound bed to have an adequate blood supply, sufficient oxygenation, healthy granulation tissue, and a supply of replicating epithelial cells, which is only possible by addressing the other components of wound bed preparation.[9] Although addressing factors that affect the epithelial edge is necessary for wound healing, the burden and pain of doing so may not be in alignment with the palliative patient's goals of care. Therefore, discuss the risks and benefits of epithelial edge advancement with the patient to determine if it is realistic to include in the plan of care. The main factors affecting epithelial edge include the following:

- Epibole, or rolled wound edges, can delay epithelial edge migration and prevent a wound from healing. Historically, the treatment of epibole is by cauterization with silver nitrate sticks, rubbing the wound edge with gauze, or surgery; however, these may not be viable options for a patient at the end of life. Some wound care products, such as the polymeric membrane dressing and the methylene blue/gentian violet dressing, are showing promise in resolving epibole, which may be an option for the palliative care patient; however, further research is needed.[21-23] Consider setting appropriate goals of care if epibole is preventing wound healing at the end of life.

- Hypergranulation tissue forms above the level of the wound margins inhibiting epithelial edge migration and stalling wound healing. The exact cause of this tissue is not known, and treatment focuses on controlling factors that are common to wounds when hypergranulation tissue begins to appear: increased exudate, infection, friction forces on the wound surface, and foreign bodies. Traditional treatment of hypergranulation tissue includes:[24]
  - o Nonselective destruction of the tissue using silver nitrate.
  - o Non-occlusive dressings applied with light pressure; foam dressings are usually the dressing of choice.
  - o Sodium chloride impregnated gauze (Mesalt® or Curasalt®).
  - o Surgical/sharp debridement of the tissue.
  - o Topical antimicrobials if infection is present.

- Undermining is an area of tissue destruction under the wound edge associated with continued exposure to shear. Undermining is often confused with tunneling, which is a tract of tissue destruction. The primary difference between undermining and tunneling is the extent of tissue destruction. Undermining involves extensive tissue destruction at the wound edge extending in multiple directions while tunneling is a small narrow tract of tissue destruction extending in one direction.[25] Areas of undermining and tunneling are loosely packed to prevent premature closure. Initiating measures to reduce shear is also necessary (*see page 41 for strategies*).

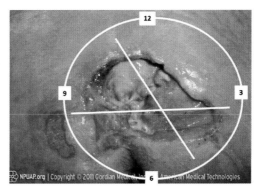

Figure 4. Example of Undermining
Photograph ©NPUAP, used with permission

- Maceration is indicative of poor exudate management. Prevent maceration using the appropriate absorptive wound care product to manage the exudate level and by applying barrier cream or liquid barrier film to the periwound tissue.[25] Induration and erythema may indicate the presence of infection or inflammation in the wound bed. Investigate these symptoms using the mnemonics NERDS and STONES (*page 19*).

KEY POINTS

- Wound bed preparation is the systematic approach of addressing wound bed characteristics that prevent healing: tissue management (debridement), inflammation/infection, moisture balance, and epithelial edge.
- Debridement is the process of removing devitalized tissue using one of five techniques – biosurgical, enzymatic, autolytic, mechanical, or sharp/surgical.
- Remember the signs and symptoms of superficial and deeper wound infections using the mnemonics NERDS and STONES.
- Select topical wound care products to manage the current level of wound exudate while minimizing the number of dressing changes.
- Epibole, hypergranulation tissue, maceration, undermining, and tunneling prevent epithelial edge migration, hindering wound healing.

References

1. Schultz GS, Sibbald RG, Falanga V, et al. Wound bed preparation: a systematic approach to wound management. *Wound Rep Reg.* 2003;11(2):1-28.

2. European Wound Management Association Position Document: *Wound Bed Preparation in Practice.* MEP Ltd, London;2004. http://www.woundsinternational.com/media/issues/87/files/content_49.pdf Accessed April 9, 2018

3. Ramundo J. Wound debridement. In Bryant RA, Nix DP, eds. *Acute & Chronic Wounds: Current Management Concepts.* 4th ed. St Louis, MO:Elsevier/Mosby;2012:279-288.

4. Burghardt J. *Wound Care Made Incredibly Visual.* 2nd ed. Ambler, PA:Lippincott Williams & Wilkins; 2011

5. Ayello EA, Cuddigan JE. Conquer chronic wounds with wound bed preparation. *Nurse Pract* 2004;29(3):8-25.

6. Santyl® collagenase ointment. Smith/Nephew; 2014. http://www.santyl.com/hcp/. Accessed April 9, 2018

7. Enzymatic Debridement with Collagenase (Santyl®). Optum Hospice Pharmacy Services. 2016. For information contact druginformation@hospiscript.com.

8. Gottrup F, Jorgensen B. Maggot debridement: alternative method for debridement. *Eplasty.* 2011;11:290-302.

9. Dowsett C, Newton H. Wound bed preparation: TIME in practice. *Wounds UK.* 2017;13(1):58-70.

10. Sibbald RG, Woo K, Ayello E. Increased bacterial burden and infection: NERDS and STONES. *Adv Skin Wound Care.* 2006:19(8):447-461 [Excerpts from this article used with permission from Wolters Kluwer Health, Inc. Copyright Clearance Center License no. 4343720866462].

11. National Pressure Ulcer Advisory Panel (NPUAP), European Pressure Ulcer Advisory Panel (EPUAP) and Pan Pacific Pressure Injury Alliance. Prevention and Treatment of Pressure Ulcers: Quick Reference Guide. Emily Haesler (Ed.). Cambridge Media: Osborne Park, Western Australia; 2014.

12. Chrisman CA. Care of chronic wounds in palliative care & end-of-life patients. *Int Wound J.* 2010;7(4);214-235.

13. Phillips PL, Wolcott RD, Fletcher J, et al. Biofilms made easy. *Wounds Intl.* 2010;1(3). http://www.woundsinternational.com/media/issues/288/files/content_8851.pdf. Accessed July 12, 2017.

14. Wolcott RD, Kennedy JP, Dowd SE. Regular debridement is the main tool for maintaining a healthy wound bed in most chronic wounds. *J Wound Care.* 2009;18(2):54-56.

15. Bradbury S, Fletcher J. Prontosan® made easy. *Wounds Intl.* 2011;2(2). https://www.bbraun.com/content/dam/catalog/bbraun/bbraunProductCatalog/S/AEM2015/en-01/b6/prontosan-made-easy.pdf.bb-.49162093/prontosan-made-easy.pdf. Accessed July 12, 2017.

16. Armstrong D, Bohn G, Glat P, et al. Expert recommendations for the use of hypochlorous acid solution: science and clinical application. *Ostomy Wound Manage.* 2015;61(5 suppl): 4S–18S.

17. Sakarya S, Gunay N, Karakulak M, et al. Hypochlorous acid: an ideal wound care agent with powerful microbicidal, antibiofilm, and wound healing potency. *Wounds.* 2014;26(12):342-350.

18. Thomas H, Wilkinson H, Stephenson C, et al. Monofilament debriding mitt reduces biofilm levels in porcine ex vivo model and in murine excisional wounds. Poster 2016 WOCN® Society & CAET Joint Conference; June 4-8, 2016; Montreal, Quebec, Canada. https://wocn.confex.com/wocn/2016am/webprogram/Paper10380.html.

19. Phillips PL, Yang Q, Sampson E, et al. Effects of antimicrobial agents on an in vitro biofilm model of skin wounds. *Adv Wound Care.* 2010;1:299-304.

20. Vowden P, Bond E, Meuleneire F. Managing high viscosity exudate. *Wounds Intl.* 2015;6(1). http://www.woundsinternational.com/media/other-resources/_/1155/files/viscous-exudate-wint.pdf. Accessed July 12, 2017.

21. Wound Source [Internet]. http://www.woundsource.com/poster/resolving-epibole-polymeric-membrane-dressings-in-home-care. Accessed April 20, 2017.

22. Benskin L. Solving the closed wound edge problem in venous ulcers using polymeric membrane dressings. Paper presented at: Wound Ostomy and Continence Nurses Society 40th Annual Conference; June 21-25, 2008; Orlando, FL. https://wocn.confex.com/wocn/2008am/techprogram/P3361.HTM. Accessed April 3, 2018.

23. Swan H, Trovela VJ. Case study review: use of an absorbent bacteriostatic dressing for multiple indications. Paper presented at: Clinical Symposium for Advances in Skin & Wound Care; September 9-11, 2011; Washington, DC. http://www.hollister.com/~/media/files/posters/alexian–bro–hfb–poster_0811.pdf. Accessed April 3, 2018.

24. Widgerow AD, Leak K. Hypergranulation tissue: evolution, control and potential elimination. *Wound Healing Southern Africa.*2010;3(2):1-3. http://www.woundhealingsa.co.za/index.php/WHSA/article/viewFile/87/127. Accessed July 11, 2017.

25. Wound, Ostomy and Continence Nurses Society (WOCN) Task Force. *Wound, Ostomy and Continence Nurses Society's guidance on OASIS-C2 integumentary items: Best practice for clinicians.* Mt. Laurel, NJ:WOCN;2016.

TOPICAL PRODUCTS FOR WOUND MANAGEMENT

GOALS

- Describe the ideal dressing for the palliative care patient
- Identify common topical products for wound management
- Become acquainted with the indications and contraindications of current wound care products

DRESSING SELECTION

Vast arrays of topical wound care products are available for use making it difficult to select an appropriate dressing. The principles of wound bed preparation assist in dressing selection. Morin and Tomaselli summarized these principles by stating:

"If a wound is desiccated, it needs to be hydrated. If a wound has excessive exudate, the fluid needs to be absorbed. If a wound has necrotic tissue or foreign debris, it needs to be debrided. Finally, if a wound is infected, it needs to be treated with an antimicrobial agent."[1]

Further expand these principles to include dead space, which is loosely packed. Additionally, evaluate other distressing wound symptoms (pruritus, odor, pain, or bleeding) and include these in the dressing selection process. Each of these situations represents an opportunity to select an ideal dressing for the conditions present in the wound at that moment.[1] For the palliative care patient, an ideal dressing would:[2]

- Be cosmetically appealing as per the patient's wishes
- Non-adhere to the wound bed
- Promote a moist wound environment
- Minimize the potential for shear or friction
- Minimize odor
- Control exudate to minimize maceration
- Have a long wear time
- Minimize pain at dressing change
- Control infection
- Be realistic for use by the patient or caregiver
- Be selected with the individualized needs or wishes of every patient

The following chart summarizes some of the currently available wound care products.

WOUND PRODUCTS CHART

Product & Description	Indications	Comments
Alginates[3,4] •Derived from brown seaweed •Forms a moisture retentive gel on contact with wound fluid •Holds up to 20x its weight in fluid *Brands: Algiderm, Algisite, Algicell, Kaltostat, CalciCare, Sorbsan, Tegagen*	•Moderate to heavy exudate (layer for increased absorption) in partial or full thickness wounds •Autolytic debridement •Packing for dead space •Odor control •Calcium alginate is hemostatic; silver alginate is antimicrobial	•Avoid use in dry wound beds, light exudate, or stable eschar •Change every 1-2 days •Requires a secondary dressing •Irrigate wound between dressing changes to remove any remaining alginate
Antibiotics, Topical[5,6] •See also *Topical Medicated Agents for Skin and Wound Care*, p112 *Brands: Neosporin, Polysporin, Bactroban*	•Bacitracin/neomycin/polymyxin B (Neosporin®) is indicated for prevention of infection in minor cuts, scrapes, or burns. Apply 1-3 times daily. •Mupirocin (Bactroban®) is indicated for skin infections and is effective against MRSA. Apply 3 times daily.	•Check patient allergies before use •Variety of OTC antibiotic preparations are available; confirm active ingredients prior to selection and use •Monitor for side effects •Routine use of a topical antibiotic is NOT recommended due to the potential for adverse reactions and antimicrobial resistance
Cadexomer Iodine[7] •Provides sustained delivery of iodine to the superficial wound bed •Highly absorbent •No known bacterial resistance •Available as an ointment, sheet dressing, or powder *Brands: Iodosorb and Iodoflex*	•Infection in a chronic, highly exudative wound •Provides broad-spectrum antimicrobial coverage – bacteria, fungi, yeasts, MRSA •Debridement and odor control	•Use caution in patients taking lithium •Contraindicated in known allergy, thyroid disorder, renal impairment •Do not use more than 50g/dose or more than 150g in a week •Side effects: redness and swelling of wound edges and "smarting" •Requires a secondary dressing •Change in color indicates need for dressing change (brown to off-white)
Charcoal[8] •Activated charcoal *Brands: Actisorb, Carbonet, CarboFlex*	•Malodorous chronic wounds •Choose a product with both an absorbent layer and a charcoal component for best odor control	•Occlusive dressing may be necessary to contain odor, change when wet •Directions for use vary based on product manufacturer
Collagen[3,4,9-11,13] •Serves as decoy for MMPs to attack to preserve the body's collagen for healing •Available as gels, alginates, sheets, or powders or with silver to provide antimicrobial properties *Brands: BIOSTEP, Promogran*	•Nonhealing wounds (NPUAP-EPUAP recommend for nonhealing Stage 3 & 4 pressure injuries) •Minimal to moderate exudate •Full thickness pressure injuries •Wounds with tunneling •Chronic, granulating wounds	•Contraindicated in sensitivity to collagen, bovine, porcine, or avian products; may be refused by vegan, Muslim, Jewish, & Hindu populations •Moisten dry wounds and debride necrotic tissue before use •Use in infection only if treated •Requires a secondary dressing
Composites[3,4,12,13] •Two or more products combined *Brands: Covaderm, DermaDress, Alldress, Telfa Island*	•Minimal to heavy exudate •Partial or full thickness wounds •Support autolytic debridement •Use as a primary or secondary dressing	•Provides a bacterial barrier, absorbs exudate, and minimizes adhesion •Requires intact periwound skin – use liquid barrier film to protect •Not for wounds with stable eschar •Some are contraindicated in infection
Contact Layers/Silicone Dressings[3,4,13] •Porous, non-adherent, silicone mesh sheets *Brands: Mepitel, PROFORE, Restore*	•Partial or full thickness wounds •Wounds with or without depth •Infected wounds – may apply topical agent over contact layer •Fluid passes through for absorption on to separate dressing	•Not recommended for dry wounds; wounds with thick, viscous exudates; wounds with tunneling or undermining •Change weekly; not intended to be changed with each dressing change •Requires a secondary dressing

Product & Description	Indications	Comments
DACC Dressings[14] •DACC = Dialkylcarbamoyl chloride •Microbes irreversibly adhere to dressing providing mechanical removal with dressing changes •Comes in gels, swabs, pads, or ribbons *Brand: Cutimed Sorbact*	•Broad-spectrum coverage against bacteria & fungi, including MRSA & VRE •Can be used for all wounds •Can be used on any level of exudate •Change dressing daily in infected wounds	•No contraindications •Creams, disinfectants, antiseptics may reduce the effectiveness of this product •Place dressing in contact with the wound bed •May require a secondary dressing
Foams[3,4,13,15] •Non-adherent, absorptive, polyurethane that wicks away drainage •Available with silver for infection and with or without an adhesive border *Brands: ALLEVYN, Biatain, HydroCell*	•Moderate to heavy exudate (non-bordered foam can be layered for increased absorption); partial or full thickness wounds with moist necrosis; deep/cavitating wounds; around tubes •May use as a primary or secondary dressing	•Not for a dry wound bed or light exudate •Not for wounds with stable eschar •Change every 1-7 days depending on amount of drainage to prevent maceration •Change daily if infection is present
Gauze[15] •Available as woven or non-woven, cotton or synthetic, sterile or non-sterile; in many forms (pads, ribbon, strips, and rolls); plain or impregnated	•Appropriate for securing a dressing and gentle wound cleansing •Impregnated gauze assists in maintaining a moist wound bed and atraumatic removal of dressings	•Plain gauze may adhere to wound bed, increase infection risk, and slow healing •Frequent dressing changes required; increased patient discomfort and increased caregiver time
Gelling Fiber Dressings[15-18] •Soft, absorbent; absorbs exudate vertically and retains the exudate *Brand: AQUACEL (Hydrofiber), Opticell*	•Moderate to heavily exudative acute or chronic wounds •Partial or full thickness wounds, pressure injuries, wounds with dead space	•Requires a secondary dressing •Available with silver for infected wounds •Can be left in place for 3 to 7 days
Gentian Violet/Methylene Blue (GV/MB)[19] •Gentian violet/methylene blue impregnated foam *Brand: Hydrofera Blue READY or Classic*	•Treatment or prevention of infection •Provides broad-spectrum antimicrobial coverage • Moderate to heavily exudative acute, traumatic, or chronic wounds	•Does not require a secondary dressing •Can be left in place for up to 7 days •Hydrofera Blue Classic®: hydration of dressing required; Hydrofera Blue READY®: no hydration required
Honey[3,4,13] •Manuka (*Leptospermum*) honey is derived from the tea tree. Medical grade honey is purified for medical use with filtration & radiation •Available as calcium alginate, hydrocolloid, paste, gel *Brand: MEDIHONEY*	•Partial or full thickness wounds •Venous & arterial ulcers, pressure injuries •Wounds with tunneling/undermining •Reduces pain, inflammation, edema, exudate, and scarring •Reduces odor •Promotes autolytic debridement	•Contraindication: hypersensitivity to honey; patients with bee sting allergies or who are allergic to bee venom should not be affected by the honey •Not recommended for dry, necrotic wounds; following incision & drainage of an abscess; wounds requiring surgical debridement •Requires a secondary dressing
Hydrocolloids[3,4,13,15] •Occlusive dressing; forms gelatinous mass to reduce wound contamination •Water resistant outer layer •Also available as a paste or powder •May use as a primary or secondary dressing *Brands: DuoDERM, Exuderm, REPLICARE*	•Minimal to moderate exudative wound with slough present •Partial or full thickness wounds without depth •Supports autolytic debridement •Maintains moist wound surface •Provides pain relief; however, may tear fragile periwound skin	•Not for infected wounds; wounds with deep tunnels, tracts, undermining, or stable eschar •Can promote infection in high-risk patients; a foul odor may develop and can be mistaken for infection •Change every 3-5 days or when fluid leaks from under wafer; dislodges with heavy exudate, shearing, or friction
Hydrogel[3,4,13,15] •Water- or glycerin-based amorphous gels, sheets or impregnated gauzes that hydrate the wound bed *Brands: PluroGel, Skintegrity*	•Dry to minimal exudate •Partial or full thickness wounds •Radiation damaged skin •Supports autolytic debridement •Adds moisture; softens necrotic tissue •Decreases pain	•Apply sheet form every 1-3 days, non-sterile gel daily, sterile gel every 3 days •Requires a secondary dressing •Prevent maceration: apply skin barrier ointment or skin sealant to intact skin •Cool sheets in refrigerator to relieve pruritus and decrease pain

Product & Description	Indications	Comments
Impregnated Gauze (sodium chloride)[20] •Available in dressings or ribbons *Brands: Mesalt, Curasalt*	•Infected wounds with moderate to heavy discharge, deep wounds, tunneling, undermining, and highly exudative wounds •Absorbs exudate, bacteria, and necrotic tissue	•Contraindicated in wounds with no or low exudate •Easy to use •Can be used to debride a highly exudative wound •Requires a secondary dressing
Impregnated Gel[21] •Hydrogel infused with sodium hypochlorite *Brand: Anasept*	•Indicated for acute and chronic infected wounds for broad-spectrum coverage: pressure injuries, diabetic foot ulcers, venous ulcers, irradiated skin, partial or full thickness wounds with no or minimal exudate	•Discontinue with any redness or irritation •Requires daily dressing changes •Requires a secondary dressing •Avoid use with silver products
Liquid Barrier Films/Liquid Skin Protectants[3,4,22] •Liquid transparent film *Brands: No Sting Skin Prep, Cavilon No Sting Barrier*	•Use around wound before applying dressing to protect surrounding skin from maceration and adhesive trauma – available as a spray, swab, or wipe	•Use non-alcohol based product for no sting application (alcohol-free products: Cavilon No Sting®, No Sting Skin Prep®) •Do NOT use around open flames – these products are extremely flammable
Moisture Wicking Fabric[23] •Fabric that wicks moisture *Brand: InterDry, Interdry Ag*	•Painful, red, inflamed skin folds with or without denuded areas	•May be worn up to 5 days •Controls moisture, odor, and inflammation of skin folds
Negative Pressure Wound Therapy[24,25] •Negative pressure to remove interstitial fluid, decrease edema, and increase blood flow	•Treatment of Stage 3 and 4 pressure injuries, chronic wounds, surgical wounds, diabetic ulcers to promote granulation and wound healing •Silver products are available	•Intermittent or continuous suction •Contraindications include fistulas to organs or body cavities, necrotic tissue, untreated osteomyelitis, malignancy, exposed blood vessels/organs •Risk of adverse events – always follow manufacturer's guidelines for use
Polyhexamethylene biguanide (PHMB)[26] •Available in sponges, rolls, gauze, and packing strips *Brands: Kerlix AMD, Curity AMD*	•Effective against Gram-negative and Gram-positive bacteria, fungi, yeast, MRSA, and VRE	•Often recommended for surgical site infection prevention •Hypoallergenic •Avoid using as a painful wet-to-dry dressing •Requires a secondary dressing
Polymeric Membrane Dressings[27] •Cleanses; fills dead space; absorbent *Brand: PolyMem*	•Any level of exudate, moisten with saline for dry wound beds •Indicated for pressure injuries, skin tears, diabetic/venous/arterial ulcers, surgical incisions, 1st or 2nd-degree burns	•Change up to every 7 days •Wound cleansing usually not required •Promotes autolytic debridement •Secure with tape or use bordered polymeric membrane dressing
Silver[28,29] •Provides broad-spectrum antimicrobial coverage – Gram-negative and positive bacteria, fungi, yeasts, MRSA, VRE, and viruses •Available in a variety of products: foams, alginates, fibers, pastes, powders, specialty absorptives, contact layers, hydrogels, fillers *Brands: AQUACEL Ag, Arglaes Powder, Mepilex Ag, PolyMem Silver, Silverlon*	•Wounds with localized, spreading, or systemic infection, including burns, surgical incisions, or chronic wounds •As a barrier for any wound, acute or chronic, at high risk of developing an infection •Select based on exudate level – if highly exudative, use an absorptive product; if dry, use a product that donates moisture •Cleanse with sterile water with some silver dressings [e.g., Silverlon® (normal saline reduces release of silver ions)]	•Contraindications: acute wounds with low infection risks, chronic wound that is healing, concurrent use with enzymatic debridement, allergy/sensitivity to silver, patients undergoing MRI or radiation therapy (per manufacturer's instruction) •Use for two weeks only and reassess: *Improving* – continue use *Infection resolved* –select new dressing *Unchanged* – select new antimicrobial •Requires a secondary dressing

Product & Description	Indications	Comments
Specialty Absorptives[30] •High absorptive capacity, semi-adherent or non-adherent *Brands: Drawtex (Hydroconductive dressing), Cutisorb Ultra, Exu-dry*	•Any heavily exudative wound to manage exudate and reduce frequency of dressing changes	•Multilayer products •May use as a primary or secondary dressing
Tapes[31] •Acrylic adhesives: adhesion increases with wear time •Silicone adhesives: adhesion does not increase with wear time	•Use acrylic adhesives to secure critical tubing/equipment, borders of dressing products •Use silicone adhesives in patients with fragile skin	•Remove all tape slowly •Liquid barrier film may prevent epidermal stripping from tape removal •Never stretch or apply tension to tape during application
Transparent Films[3,4] •Occlusive, non-absorbent dressings; permeable to oxygen and water vapor, impermeable to bacteria/contaminants *Brands: Opsite, Suresite, Tegaderm*	•Dry to minimal exudate, shallow or partial thickness wounds •Supports autolytic debridement •Maintains moist wound surface •Protects from friction, shear, microbes, and chemicals	•Not for exudative or infected wounds •Need 2-inch border around wound •Change every 3-7 days or if exudate is beyond wound border •May use as a primary or secondary dressing
Wound Cleansers[3,4] •Normal saline: primary cleanser; use fresh solution daily •Commercial wound cleanser: contains surfactants to loosen and lift debris *Brands: Allclenz, Carraklenz, Skintegrity*	•Cleansing with each dressing change removes surface bacteria & debris •Clean wound bed: pour normal saline or wound cleanser •Infection/necrosis: irrigate with wound cleanser or antiseptic	•Switch to commercial wound cleanser or antiseptic if infection is present •Irrigate with 4-15 psi: piston syringe (4.2 psi), squeeze bottle with irrigation cap (4.5 psi), or 35 mL syringe and 18 gauge needle (8 psi)
Antiseptic Cleansers*		
Acetic Acid[3,4,32] •Acetic Acid (0.25, 0.5%)	•Antibacterial and antifungal properties •Effective against *Pseudomonas aeruginosa* •Use as a soak for superficial wounds	•Use may result in overgrowth of unsusceptible bacteria •May cause pain with use •Frequent application needed
Povidone-iodine[33] •Betadine® (5, 7.5, 10, 15%)	•Broad-spectrum against bacteria, fungi, and viruses •Maximum dose is TID for 7 days	•Assess for patient allergies before use •Do not apply to large areas •Caution in patients with burns, renal insufficiency, and thyroid disorders
Sodium Hypochlorite Solution[34] •Dakin's® solution 0.5% full, 0.25% half, 0.125% quarter, 0.0125% Di-Dak-Sol®	•Broad-spectrum coverage •Indicated for prevention and treatment of wound infections •Activity against Gram-negative bacteria, MRSA	•Short-term therapy (≤ 14 days) •Apply daily or twice daily •If not commercially prepared, discard unused solution after 24 hours •Use as a wet-to-moist dressing twice daily for debridement
Hydrogen Peroxide	•Cytotoxic; avoid use in wound care.	

Wound Fillers[3,4]
•Dressing materials placed into open wounds to eliminate dead space
 	
Brands: DuoDERM Hydroactive Paste, PolyMem Wic, FLEXIGEL Strands
	•Appropriate for
	  •minimal to moderate exudates
	  •full thickness wounds with depth
	  •infected or non-infected wounds
	  •wounds with dead space
		•Use appropriate secondary dressing to optimize moist wound environment
		•Change dressing every 1-2 days
		•Available as hydrated pastes or gels; dry powder, granules, or beads; or as cavity dressings, ropes, or pillows

Wound Manager Pouches[36]
•Pouches placed over highly exudative wounds, fistulas, or multiple stomas
 	
Brands: Eakin Wound Pouch, Hollister Wound Drainage Collector Pouch
	•Appropriate for
	  •Fistulas
	  •Stomas – multiple or irregularly shaped
	  •Highly exudative wounds
		•Improve patient comfort and reduce patient care time
		•Can be emptied, connected to drainage collector, or suction

*The FDA has ruled 24 active ingredients of health care antiseptics are not generally recommended as safe and effective (GRASE). The primary ingredients affected by this ruling is triclosan and chlorhexidine gluconate. Until additional data is received, the FDA deferred ruling for one year on 6 active ingredients of health care antiseptics: benzalkonium chloride, benzethonium chloride, chloroxylenol, alcohol, isopropyl alcohol, and povidone-iodine. Additional information at reference 35

USING WOUND CONDITION TO ASSIST IN PRODUCT SELECTION

Using Wound Condition to Assist in Product Selection	
Wound Bed Characteristic	**Possible Treatment Options**
Biofilm[37-43] *Thin, slimy layer of bacteria that adheres to surface of wound bed. May cause signs/symptoms of superficial infection and delayed wound healing.*	*Select one approach:* • Irrigate and soak (for 3-5 minutes) wound with betaine and polyhexanide (PHMB) surfactant (Prontosan®) or hypochlorous acid solution (Vashe® Wound Therapy Solution/ Dakin solution). Apply an antimicrobial dressing. • Apply PHMB viscous gel (Prontosan® gel) as primary dressing and change daily. • Impregnate primary dressing with hypochlorous acid solution (Vashe® Wound Therapy Solution/Solution). • Apply cadexomer iodine (Iodosorb® – effective against *Pseudomonas aeruginosa*).
Dead Space *A cavity in the wound bed. Loosely fill the wound cavity to prevent premature closure.*	• **None or minimal exudate:** Loosely pack hydrogel impregnated gauze into the wound bed, cover with a composite dressing or transparent film. • **Moderate or heavy exudate:** Loosely pack calcium alginate or a gelling fiber dressing (Hydrofiber®) into the wound bed, cover with a bordered foam dressing.
Dry Wound Bed *Wound bed lacking exudate. A moist wound bed promotes granulation, re-epithelialization, and autolysis while reducing cell death and pain.*	• Wound of any thickness: Apply polymeric membrane dressing moistened with saline. • Partial thickness wound (goal is to *retain* moisture): Apply transparent film or hydrocolloid. • Full thickness wound (goal is to *add* moisture): Apply hydrogel to wound bed and cover with a composite dressing or transparent film.
Epibole[44-46] *Rolled wound edge. Epibole prevents re-epithelialization.*	• Polymeric membrane dressings applied with pressure to the wound edge. • Gentian violet/methylene blue (GV/MB) dressings. Change per manufacturer's recommendation.
Epithelializing *New epithelial cells, pink in color.*	• Protect by applying hydrocolloid, transparent film, or foam to wound bed.
Stable Eschar[47-50] *Black, leathery necrotic tissue firmly adhered to wound bed. No drainage or odor.*	• Paint the perimeter of the wound with povidone-iodine or chlorhexidine daily and leave open to air. Protect with gauze/clean sock as needed. • Debridement only if healing is the goal: Apply hydrogel, cover with clear film dressing. *Do NOT debride dry, stable eschar present on heels or elbows.*
Granulation Tissue *Red, bumpy tissue comprised of collagen and new blood vessels.*	• Apply hydrocolloid, polymeric membrane dressing, transparent film, or non-adherent foam to wound bed. Cover with a secondary dressing if needed.
Hypergranulation Tissue[51] *Granulation tissue above the level of the wound margins. Prevents re-epithelialization.*	*Select either:* • Apply foam dressing with slight compression • Apply sodium chloride impregnated gauze (Mesalt®), cover with a composite dressing. Rule out infection and malignancy.
Infection *Superficial (NERDS) and deeper (STONES) infections delay healing and reduce quality of life.*[52]	• **None or minimal exudate:** Apply silver hydrogel, cover with an island composite dressing. • **Moderate or heavy exudate:** Apply silver alginate or a gelling fiber dressing with silver (Hydrofiber® with silver), cover with a bordered foam dressing.
Maceration *White, softened periwound skin from excess exudate.*	• Apply liquid barrier film or barrier cream to periwound tissue with each dressing change. • Use a more absorbent dressing, rule out infection.
Slough/Necrotic Tissue *Devitalized tissue in the wound bed, may be yellow, grey, tan, brown, or green. Loosely or firmly adherent to wound bed. Various levels of moisture.*	• **None or minimal exudate:** Apply hydrogel to wound bed, cover with a composite dressing or transparent film. *Alternatively,* apply a hydrocolloid. • **Moderate exudate:** Apply calcium alginate, cover with a bordered foam dressing. • **Heavy exudate:** Apply a gelling fiber dressing (Hydrofiber®), cover with a bordered foam dressing. *Alternatively,* apply sodium chloride impregnated gauze (Mesalt®), cover with a composite dressing.

KEY POINTS

- No definitive research is available to guide the selection of one product over another.
- Match the characteristics of the wound to the indications and contraindications of the dressing provided in the manufacturer's guidelines.
- For the palliative care patient, address distressing symptoms, including pain, odor, exudate, and cosmetic appeal, during the dressing selection process.

References

1. Morin RJ, Tomaselli NL. Dressings and topical agents. *Clin Plastic Surg*. 2007;34:643-658.
2. Chrisman CA. Care of chronic wounds in palliative care and end-of-life patients. *Int Wound J*. 2010;7:214-235.
3. Burghardt J. Wound Care Made Incredibly Visual. 2nd ed. Ambler, PA:Lippincott Williams & Wilkins; 2011.
4. Bryant RA, Nix DP, eds. *Acute & Chronic Wounds: Current Management Concepts*. 4th ed. St Louis, MO:Elsevier/Mosby; 2012.
5. Bacitracin (topical). Lexi-Drugs Online. Lexicomp. Wolters Kluwer; Hudson, OH. Accessed April 16, 2018
6. Mupirocin. Lexi-Drugs Online. Lexicomp. Wolters Kluwer; Hudson, OH. Accessed April 16, 2018
7. Iodine (Iodosorb). Lexi-Drugs Online. Lexicomp. Wolters Kluwer; Hudson, OH. Accessed April 16, 2018
8. Thomas S, Fisher B, Fram P, et al. Odour absorbing dressings: a comparative laboratory study. *World Wide Wounds*. 1998(1). http://www.worldwidewounds.com/1998/march/Odour-Absorbing-Dressings/odour-absorbing-dressings.html. Accessed June 13, 2017.
9. Wound care dressings: collagens. Wound Care Education Institute. https://blog.wcei.net/tag/collagen-dressings. Accessed June 13, 2017.
10. Morgan N. What you need to know about collagen dressings. Wound Care Advisor. https://woundcareadvisor.com/what-you-need-to-know-about-collagen-wound-dressings/. Accessed June 13, 2017.
11. National Pressure Ulcer Advisory Panel (NPUAP), European Pressure Ulcer Advisory Panel (EPUAP) and Pan Pacific Pressure Injury Alliance. Prevention and Treatment of Pressure Ulcers: Quick Reference Guide. Emily Haesler (Ed.). Cambridge Media: Osborne Park, Western Australia; 2014.
12. WoundSource: Composites. Wound Source; Kestrel Health Information. Available at http://www.woundsource.com/product-category/dressings/composites. Accessed April 20, 2017.
13. Wounds 360. Wounds360 Product Guide. Available at http://www.wounds360bg.com/ Accessed April 6, 2018.
14. Totty J, Bua N, Smith G, et al. Dialkylcarbamoyl chloride (DACC)-coated dressings in the management and prevention of wound infection. *J Wound Care* 2017;26(3):107-114
15. Sood A, Granick MS, Tomaselli NL. Wound dressings and comparative effectiveness data. *Adv Wound Care*. 2014;3(8):511-529.
16. Hydrofiber technology: Aquacel. ConvaTec, Inc. https://www.convatec.com/wound-skin/aquacel-dressings/hydrofiber-technology/ Accessed April 20, 2017.
17. Baranoski S. Wound & skin care: choosing a wound dressing, part 2. *Nursing*. 2008;38(2):14-15.
18. Barnea Y, Weiss J, Gur E. A review of the applications of the hydrofiber dressing with silver (Aquacel Ag®) in wound care. *Ther Clin Risk Manag*. 2010;6:21-27.
19. Hydrofera Blue. Hollister; 2014. Available at http://www.hollister.com/~/media/files/pdfs–for–download/wound–care/hydroferablue-ready-brochure-922496-0214.pdf. Accessed February 6, 2018.
20. Mesalt. Molnlycke. Available at http://www.molnlycke.us/advanced-wound-care-products/alginates-debriders-gels/mesalt/. Accessed April 20, 2017.
21. Anasept antimicrobial skin & wound gel. Anacapa Tech. Available at http://anacapa-tech.net/product/anasept-antimicrobial-skin-wound-gel/anasept-antimicrobial-skin-wound-gel-2/ Accessed April 19, 2017.
22. Barrier film: product use directions. 3M Health Care Division; 2004. Available at http://multimedia.3m.com/mws/media/490989O/cavilon-no-sting-barrier-film-product-use-directions.pdf Accessed June 13, 2017.

23. WoundSource. InterDry moisture wicking fabric with antimicrobial silver. Wound Source; Kestrel Health Information. Available at http://www.woundsource.com/product/interdry-moisture-wicking-fabric-antimicrobial-silver Accessed June 13, 2017.

24. Netsch DS. Negative pressure wound therapy. In Bryant RA, Nix DP, eds. *Acute & Chronic Wounds: Current Management Concepts.* 4th ed. St Louis, MO:Elsevier/Mosby;2012:337-344.

25. Gestring M. Negative pressure wound therapy. In: Post T, ed. *UpToDate*, Waltham, MA: *UpToDate*;2018. Accessed April 16, 2018.

26. Kirker K, Fisher S, James G, et al. Efficacy of polyhexamethylene biguanide-containing antimicrobial foam dressing against MRSA relative to standard foam dressing. *Wounds* 2009; 21(9): 229-233

27. PolyMem. Ferris Mfg Corp; Available at http://www.polymem.com/ Accessed May 1, 2017.

28. Leaper D. Appropriate use of silver dressings in wounds: international consensus document. *Int Wound J* 2012;9(5):461-464

29. Friedman C, Bass E, Steinberg J. Key considerations for utilizing silver dressings. *Podiatry Today.* 2006;19(6). http://www.podiatrytoday.com/article/5530. Accessed April 18, 2017.

30. WoundSource: Specialty Absorptives/Super Absorbents. Wound Source; Kestrel Health Information. Available at http://www.woundsource.com/product-category/dressings/specialty-absorptives. Accessed April 20, 2017.

31. Taroc AM. Guide for adhesive removal: principles, practices, and products. *American Nurse Today.* 2017; 12(10):24-26

32. Acetic Acid, Glacial. Clinical Pharmacology. Gold Standard, Inc. Accessed April 16 2018

33. Povidone-Iodine. Clinical Pharmacology. Gold Standard, Inc. Accessed April 16 2018

34. Dakins quarter (sodium hypochlorite solution). [Package insert]. Century Pharmaceuticals, Inc Available https://dailymed.nlm.nih.gov/dailymed/drugInfo.cfm?setid=9906e5fe-7bf5-4d99-8107-c048bb5e42d5

35. Food & Drug Administration (FDA). Safety and effectiveness of health care antiseptics; topical antimicrobial drug products for over-the-counter human use. Final Rule. *Fed Regist* 2017;82(243):60474-60503 Available https://www.gpo.gov/fdsys/pkg/FR-2017-12-20/pdf/2017-27317.pdf Accessed April 16 2018

36. Wound pouches. Eakin. Available at http://www.eakin.eu/professional-wound-pouches. Accessed August 8, 2017.

37. Phillips PL, Wolcott RD, Fletcher J, et al. Biofilms made easy. *Wounds Intl.* 2010;1(3). http://www.woundsinternational.com/media/issues/288/files/content_8851.pdf. Accessed July 12, 2017.

38. Wolcott RD, Kennedy JP, Dowd SE. Regular debridement is the main tool for maintaining a healthy wound bed in most chronic wounds. *J Wound Care.* 2009;18(2):54-56.

39. Bradbury S, Fletcher J. Prontosan® made easy. *Wounds Intl.* 2011;2(2). https://www.bbraun.com/content/dam/catalog/bbraun/bbraunProductCatalog/S/AEM2015/en-01/b6/prontosan-made-easy.pdf.bb-.49162093/prontosan-made-easy.pdf. Accessed July 12, 2017.

40. Armstrong D, Bohn G, Glat P, et al. Expert recommendations for the use of hypochlorous acid solution: science and clinical application. *Ostomy Wound Manage.* 2015;61(5 suppl): 4S–18S.

41. Sakarya S, Gunay N, Karakulak M, et al. Hypochlorous acid: an ideal wound care agent with powerful microbicidal, antibiofilm, and wound healing potency. *Wounds.* 2014;26(12):342-350.

42. Thomas H, Wilkinson H, Stephenson C, et al. Monofilament debriding mitt reduces biofilm levels in porcine ex vivo model and in murine excisional wounds. Poster presented at: 2016 WOCN® Society & CAET Joint Conf; June 4-8, 2016; Montreal, Quebec, Canada. https://wocn.confex.com/wocn/2016am/webprogram/Paper10380.html.

43. Phillips PL, Yang Q, Sampson E, et al. Effects of antimicrobial agents on an in vitro biofilm model of skin wounds. *Adv Wound Care.* 2010;1:299-304.

44. Bare K, Drain J. Resolving epibole with polymeric membrane dressings in home care. WoundSource Online Poster Hall. Available at http://www.woundsource.com/poster/resolving-epibole-polymeric-membrane-dressings-in-home-care Accessed April 16, 2018.

45. Benskin L. Solving the closed wound edge problem in venous ulcers using polymeric membrane dressings. *J Wound Ostomy Continence Nurs* 2008;35(3):S30-S31.

46. Swan H, Trovela VJ. Case study review: use of an absorbent bacteriostatic dressing for multiple indications. Clinical Symposium for Advances in Skin & Wound Care; September 9-11, 2011; Washington, DC. http://www.hollister.com/~/media/files/posters/alexian–bro–hfb–poster_0811.pdf Accessed April 3, 2018.

47. Wound Ostomy and Continence Nurses Society. A quick reference guide for lower-extremity wounds: venous, arterial, and neuropathic. 2013 http://c.ymcdn.com/sites/www.wocn.org/resource/collection/E3050C1A-FBF0-44ED-B28B-C41E24551CCC/A_Quick_Reference_Guide_for_LE_Wounds_(2013).pdf. Accessed July 14, 2017.

48. Wound Ostomy and Continence Nurses Society. Guideline for management of wounds in patients with lower-extremity arterial disease. AHRQ;2014. https://www.guideline.gov/summaries/summary/49162/guideline-for-management-of-wounds-in-patients-with-lowerextremity-arterial-disease?q=arterial+ulcers. Accessed July 14, 2017.
49. Takahashi P. Chronic ischemic, venous, and neuropathic ulcers in long-term care. *Ann LTC.* 2006;14(7):26-31.
50. Williams RL. Cadexomer iodine: an effective palliative dressing in chronic critical limb ischemia. *Wounds.* 2009;21(1):15-28
51. Widgerow AD, Leak K. Hypergranulation tissue: evolution, control and potential elimination. *Wound Healing Southern Africa.*2010;3(2):1-3. http://www.woundhealingsa.co.za/index.php/WHSA/article/viewFile/87/127. Accessed July 11, 2017.
52. Sibbald RG, Woo K, Ayello E. Increased bacterial burden and infection: NERDS and STONES. *Adv Skin Wound Care.* 2006:19(8):447-461

PRESSURE INJURY PREVENTION AND TREATMENT

GOALS

Within the confines of the patient's prognosis and in alignment with the wishes of the patient and family:

- Maintain skin integrity with individualized prevention strategies
- Provide localized wound care that maintains a moist wound bed, minimizes the risk of developing an infection, and promotes quality of life
- Ensure wound care interventions relieve distressing symptoms, such as pain, odor, and exudate

DEFINITIONS

A **pressure injury** is an area of skin or underlying tissue damage usually associated with a bony prominence or under a medical device. The injury is the result of an extended period of pressure to the area or from a combination of pressure and shear. The extent of the damage can range from intact skin with non-blanchable erythema to full thickness ulcerations with exposed muscle or bone. Pain frequently accompanies these injuries. In the palliative care patient, risk factors for the development of a pressure injury include immobility, excessive moisture, shear from bed mobility activities, co-morbidities, and nutritional deficiencies.[1]

The use of medical devices, such as oxygen delivery devices, rectal tubes, or nasogastric tubes, can lead to the development of pressure injuries. Pressure injuries found on the mucous membranes as a result of pressure from a medical device are called **mucosal membrane pressure injuries.** It is NOT appropriate to stage these injuries. Pressure injuries due to medical devices found in other areas of the body (excluding mucous membranes) are called **device-related pressure injuries**. Stage these pressure injuries using the staging criteria provided below.[1]

Reverse staging is the practice of referring to healing pressure injuries in reverse order; however, reverse staging is not an accurate representation of the healing process. Once layers of tissue and supporting structures are gone, such as with full thickness wounds, they are not replaced. Instead, granulation tissue fills the wound bed. Consequently, a Stage 3 pressure injury cannot progress to a Stage 1 or 2. Describe a Stage 3 pressure injury that is granulating as a healing Stage 3 pressure injury.[2]

Within the regulatory environment of long-term care, pressure injuries are classified as avoidable or unavoidable. **Avoidable pressure injuries** are those that arise from facility failure to accurately assess patient risk factors and implement, monitor, and revise interventions based on the patient's assessment. **Unavoidable pressure injuries** are just the opposite. The facility provided the standard of care necessary to prevent a pressure injury, but a pressure injury still developed. The development of an unavoidable pressure injury can be related to the patient's declining health status at the end of life. Documentation or lack thereof can also differentiate an avoidable from an unavoidable pressure injury. Therefore, thoroughly document on all interventions, the patient's response to these interventions, and any revisions to the plan of the care.[3]

ASSESSMENT

Complete a skin and wound assessment to identify the patient's risk for pressure injuries, and to document existing skin injury.[4] Refer to page 7 for suggestions regarding the completion and documentation of a skin and wound assessment. One component of the assessment is identifying the stage of the pressure injury. The following reflects the latest pressure injury staging guidelines from the National Pressure Ulcer Advisory Panel.[1]

Pressure Injury Stages[1]

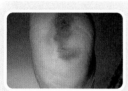

Deep Tissue Pressure Injury

- Intact or open skin
- May present as non-blanchable skin (dark red, maroon, purple); dark wound bed; or *blood*-filled blister
- May deteriorate to reveal extensive tissue loss or may resolve without a loss of tissue

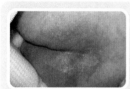

Stage 1

- Intact skin with non-blanchable redness
- Should NOT see dark red, maroon or purple areas (this is a deep tissue pressure injury)

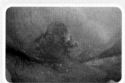

Stage 2

- May present as: partial thickness tissue loss with exposed dermis and a pink or red wound bed; or as an intact or broken *serum*-filled blister
- Should NOT see granulation tissue, slough, eschar, adipose tissue, muscle, bone, or tendon

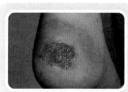

Stage 3

- Full thickness ulceration; adipose tissue is visible
- Can see slough, eschar, or granulation tissue
- Epibole, undermining, and tunneling are possible
- Should NOT see muscle, tendon, or bone

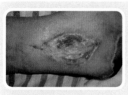

Stage 4

- Full thickness ulceration; fascia, muscle, tendon, ligament, cartilage, or bone is visible or palpable
- Can see slough, eschar, or granulation tissue
- Epibole, undermining, and tunneling are possible

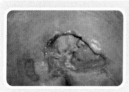

Unstageable

- Full thickness ulceration
- Depth unknown because it is obscured by slough or eschar
- Debridement will reveal either a Stage 3 or Stage 4 pressure injury

Photographs ©NPUAP, used with permission

A risk assessment tool identifies patients at risk of developing a pressure injury and allows for proactive placement of preventive interventions. Use the risk assessment tool in conjunction with clinical judgment to identify patients that would benefit from prevention strategies. Multiple risk assessment tools are available for use. One of the most widely used risk assessment tools is *The Braden Scale for Predicting Pressure Sore Risk*. The Braden Scale assesses risk in six areas: sensory perception, skin moisture, activity, mobility, nutrition, and friction/shear. Patients are scored from 'at risk' to 'very high risk' for the development of pressure injuries with scores ranging from 6 to 23. Increase preventive strategies as the patient's risk of developing a pressure injury increases. A score of 9 or less is very high risk and requires the most extensive preventive measures. Typically, this scale is used for patients in the acute care, home care, or long-term care setting.[5]

In palliative care, a few risk assessment tools are available (*see page 119*). The Hunters Hill Marie Curie Centre pressure sore risk assessment tool is specifically for the palliative care population. This tool assesses pressure injury risk in seven areas: sensation, mobility, moisture, bed mobility, nutrition/weight changes, skin condition, and friction/shear.[6] Limitations of this tool include the lack of a 'no risk' category and differentiation of 'high risk' versus 'very high risk'.[7] The Hospice Pressure Ulcer Risk Assessment Scale (HoRT scale) is a simplified tool for the palliative care population. This tool evaluates three areas: physical activity, mobility, and age. Although further evaluation of this scale is needed, it has shown promise in its ability to identify at risk patients.[8]

Best Practices for Pressure Injury Prevention – Assessment[4-9]

- Complete a comprehensive assessment of the patient upon admission. Include:
    - Head to toe assessment, including current assessment of skin and any wounds, with emphasis on any signs or symptoms that would indicate a change in condition
    - Level of pain using an appropriate pain scale
    - Palliative Performance Scale (PPS) score
    - Stage of existing pressure injuries
    - Patient's goals of care and impact of pressure injury care and/or prevention strategies on quality of life
    - Current caregiver situation:
        - Ability to provide skin care and assist with mobility
        - Ability to provide increased care as the patient's condition declines
    - Risk Assessment (should be completed within 8 hours of admission if inpatient)
        - The Braden Scale for Predicting Pressure Sore Risk©
        - Hunters Hill Marie Curie Centre pressure sore risk assessment – for palliative care
    - Contributing Factors Assessment
        - The palliative care population is at high-risk of pressure injury development due to multiple intrinsic and extrinsic factors (*see page 6*)
    - Assess healing using the Pressure Ulcer Scale for Healing (PUSH©) if healing is the goal
- Repeat the comprehensive assessment regularly as defined by organizational policies
- Educate the patient on all assessment findings and possible prevention strategies
- Customize the care plan based upon the wishes of and the risk factors identified for the patient

PLAN OF CARE

Develop an individualized plan of care to prevent and treat pressure injuries, if present, to guide the actions of all members of the interdisciplinary team. The care plan serves to translate the data gained from completion of the comprehensive assessment and risk assessment into a specific plan of action for all members of the care team. Table 1 reviews potential care plans for pressure injuries.[10]

Table 1. Care Plans for Pressure Injuries[10]		
Nursing Diagnosis	Related Factors	Interventions
Risk for Impaired Skin Integrity • Patient has the potential for an alteration in skin integrity	• Potential for/existence of prolonged, unrelieved pressure • Shearing • Altered sensation or circulation • Immobility • Moisture • Medications • Knowledge deficit • Inadequate nutrition	• Assess skin, note areas of discoloration, texture, or temperature and any existing skin alterations • Turn and reposition (state frequency) • Provide pressure-redistributing surface • Assist with bed mobility and transfers • Maintain skin clean and dry • Provide incontinence care • Preventive dressings to bony prominences • Maximize nutritional status when appropriate • Increase activity, if able • Assess skin alteration and determine etiology • Localized wound care, monitor daily
Impaired Skin Integrity • Partial thickness tissue loss		
Impaired Tissue Integrity • Full thickness tissue loss		

INTERVENTIONS

Activity, Mobility
Limitations in mobility and activity are prerequisite risk factors for the development of a pressure injury. If the patient does not have a limitation in mobility and activity, other risk factors alone should not contribute to the development of a pressure injury. Therefore, improving a patient's activity and mobility will decrease or eliminate the patient's potential for pressure injury development.[4] Typical interventions for improving activity and mobility include repositioning the patient, encouraging or assisting the patient to get out of bed or to ambulate, teaching the patient to make small shifts in their position throughout the day, and providing assistive devices to improve ambulation or bed mobility.

Patient immobility is possible at the end of life.[11] Offloading pressure is vital for the immobile patient because it creates an environment that enhances soft tissue viability, prevents the development of new pressure injuries, and promotes healing of existing pressure injuries. Common interventions to offload pressure include:[4,12]

- *Repositioning*: Shift and adjust patient position at least every 2 hours if on a regular mattress or every 4 hours if on a pressure-redistributing mattress if in alignment with the patient's wishes. Pillows or foam wedges keep bony prominences from direct contact with one another. Always assess and treat for pain if repositioning causes discomfort to the patient.
- *Pressure relief for heels*: "Float the heels" by placing a pillow longitudinally under the calves of the bedbound patient to keep the heels suspended in air. Heel protection devices that completely float the heel are also effective. Note that heel pillows ("moon boots") do not relieve pressure on the heels. These products reduce friction only.

- *Side-lying position:* When the patient is positioned on his side, avoid positioning directly on the trochanter.
- *Position the head of bed*: Maintain head of the bed at the lowest degree of elevation medically necessary to minimize shear and friction.
- *Lifting devices:* Use of lift sheets will reduce shear and friction when repositioning the patient.
- *Pressure from sitting:* At risk patients should move at least every hour. If possible, the patient should be taught to shift weight every 15 minutes.

For the patient that has limited mobility and activity, the use of pressure-redistributing support surfaces can augment other interventions to prevent consequences of immobility and are often the first intervention to prevent development or progression of pressure injuries;[11] however, support surfaces alone neither prevent nor heal pressure injuries, and they cannot replace the basic patient care practices of encouraging or assisting with ambulation and repositioning, turning and transferring. Schedule these interventions, if necessary, to ensure the routine occurs. If patient ambulation or repositioning is impossible, difficult, or painful, use of the appropriate support surfaces is critical.[13] These devices include mattresses, overlays, and cushions. Device selection will depend on the unique factors of the patient, which may include mobility, ambulatory status, microclimate, risk level, or patient preference. All support surfaces should meet the following criteria:[13]

- minimize pressure, shear, and friction while controlling moisture and temperature
- constructed with cleanable surface to minimize contamination
- compatible with multiple surfaces
- cost-effective
- address patient safety and comfort

Support surfaces fall into several categories:[14]

- **Reactive Support Surface** – provides pressure redistribution by conforming to body contours. Includes powered and non-powered overlays and mattresses of foam, air, or viscous fluid.
- **Active Support Surface** – provides pressure redistribution by alternating contact with the body at set intervals. Includes powered overlays and mattresses of air.
- **Non-powered** – Does not require an external energy source to operate.
- **Powered** – Requires an external energy source to operate.
- **Integrated Bed System** – A single unit bed frame and support surface.
- **Low Air Loss** – A feature of a support surface that enhances microclimate by increasing evaporation from the patient's skin. Used to manage moisture.
- **Alternating Pressure** – A feature of a support surface that changes pressure to an area of the body by alternating high and low pressures.

Selecting an appropriate support surface for the patient is essential. Deciding upon an appropriate support surface is often up to the discretion of the clinician and rarely on evidence-based practice.[15,16] Use the following table to assist in selecting an appropriate mattress or overlay support surface. This table applies to patients with an existing pressure injury (excluding pressure injuries of the heels) or who are at risk of developing a pressure injury, as evidenced by a Braden score ≤ 18. For patients who are not at risk of developing a pressure injury, as evidenced by a Braden score ≥ 18, use the current support surface in place, and monitor skin and Braden score regularly to determine any change that would warrant the use of a support surface.[15] Before placing any patient on a support surface, review the patient's medical record for precautions or contraindications to the use of support surfaces, such as:[15]

- Patient exceeds weight limit
- Unstable fractures of the spine
- Agitation or combativeness
- Home environment is unable to support the surface

Support Surface Selection for Patients with Existing Pressure Injuries or Braden Score ≤ 18[5,15-18]					
		Mobility (As Defined by Braden Scale)			
Guide to Support Surface Selection		**No Limitation** • Independent	**Slightly Limited** • Frequent, slight changes in position	**Very Limited** • Infrequent, slight position changes	**Immobile** • Assistance needed for all positioning
Microclimate (As Defined by Braden Scale)	**Rarely Moist** • Skin is usually dry	• Reactive foam • Static gel or air	• Reactive foam • Static gel or air	• Reactive foam • Static gel or air • Alternating pressure	• Reactive foam • Static gel or air • Alternating pressure
	Occasionally Moist • Skin sometimes moist	• Reactive foam • Static gel or air	• Reactive foam • Static gel or air	• Reactive foam • Static gel or air • Alternating pressure	• Reactive foam • Static gel or air • Alternating pressure
	Very Moist • Skin is usually moist	• Reactive foam • Static gel or air • Low air loss	• Reactive foam • Static gel or air • Low air loss	• Low air loss	• Low air loss
	Constantly Moist • Skin is always moist	• Reactive foam • Static gel or air • Low air loss	• Reactive foam • Static gel or air • Low air loss	• Low air loss • Air fluidized*	• Low air loss • Air fluidized*
*Use in the treatment of pressure injuries, not prevention					

To prevent pressure injuries in patients who spend the majority of their time in a seated position, use pressure-redistributing cushions. Keep these cushions in good repair, and ensure they facilitate a microclimate (temperature and humidity/moisture level of the skin at the support surface interface) that discourages pressure injury development. If pressure injuries develop or worsen despite the use of a pressure-redistributing cushion, consult a seating specialist, such as an Occupational Therapist, or trial a period of bed rest to relieve pressure. Donut cushions do not redistribute pressure and cause pressure injuries. Never use donut cushions to relieve pressure.[4]

Best Practices for Pressure Injury Prevention – Activity and Mobility[4]

- Pressure-Redistributing Devices:
    - Use a support surface that matches the patient's needs. Consider: bed mobility, ambulatory status, current pressure injury, risk level for developing a pressure injury, height/weight, microclimate, potential for shear, care setting
    - Reassess the need for and the function of the support surface at every visit
    - Use incontinence products, clothing, repositioning devices, and linens sparingly and only if they are compatible with the support surface
    - Consider changing the support surface if an existing pressure injury stalls or deteriorates
    - Use a pressure-redistributing seat cushion to prevent pressure injuries when seated
- Repositioning:
    - Provide assistive devices to promote activity, mobility, and independence
    - In palliative care, attempt to reposition the individual every two (regular mattress) to four (on a pressure-redistributing mattress) hours if in alignment with the patient's wishes
    - Assist or encourage the patient to reposition self at least hourly when seated
    - Create a repositioning schedule unique to the needs of the patient
    - Monitor patient's skin with each change in position
    - Avoid repositioning patients on existing pressure injuries
    - Refrain from elevating the head of bed greater than 30° unless medically required
    - Pre-medicate prior to position changes to alleviate pain with movement
    - Document attempts to turn and reposition as well as the patient's response or wishes, including the desire to maintain a position of comfort
- Medical Devices:
    - Remove bedpans immediately after use
    - Never position a patient on a medical device
- Heels:
    - Float heels so that they are free from the bed surface
    - For Stage 1 or 2 heel pressure injuries: float heels using a pillow or heel suspension device
    - For Stage 3, 4, or unstageable heel pressure injuries: use a heel suspension device

Manage Moisture

Skin, when exposed to urine, stool, perspiration, or wound exudate, is at an increased risk of experiencing breakdown, such as maceration. Maceration weakens collagen fibers and skin resilience, especially in the presence of mechanical forces (e.g., friction, tape removal, pressure) or chemical agents (e.g., harsh skin cleansers, GI secretions, stool).[19] Also, wet or moist skin tends to adhere to bed linens, which places the patient at risk of experiencing friction and shear. Finally, wet skin is susceptible to irritation, rashes, and infection.[20] Further compounding the problem is skin exposure to liquid stool, which results in rapid skin breakdown.[19] Patients with fecal incontinence are 22 times more likely to develop pressure injuries than patients who are not incontinent of stool.[21] Use of protective barriers and moisture-absorbing products is essential. (*See Topical Medicated Agents chart on page 112 for more information*). Containment devices, such as external pouches (e.g., rectal, ostomy, perianal), indwelling catheters,[19] incontinence pads and briefs to wick moisture away from the skin, are additional methods to protect patient skin.[22,23]

Steps in a skin maintenance regimen include:[19]

1. Cleanse skin with a pH balanced cleanser as soon as it is soiled
   - Cleansing of the skin after each fecal incontinence episode is vital because briefs can trap stool against the skin.
2. Moisturize and lubricate the skin. Moisturizers may be incorporated into commercially prepared skin cleansers.
3. Apply a skin protectant (sealant, ointment, or paste) depending on need:
   - Skin sealants protect the skin from maceration but have limited effectiveness at protecting the skin from enzymes.
   - Moisture barrier ointments protect the skin from enzymes but may be inadequate if excessive moisture is present.
   - Pastes are appropriate with high-volume output or diarrhea.

Best Practices for Pressure Injury Prevention – Managing Moisture[4]
• Use a skin cleanser that is pH balanced
• Cleanse skin as soon as it is soiled
• Refrain from massaging or rubbing skin that is vulnerable to pressure injuries. This is a source of friction.
• Create an individualized program to manage incontinence
• Use barrier products to protect against moisture damage
• Moisturize the skin to maintain hydration
• Consider the use of a support surface to assist in managing microclimate

Friction and Shear

The concepts of friction and shear are a source of confusion. A notable point is the removal of friction from the definition of pressure injury to prevent the diagnosis of friction injuries as pressure injuries. Injuries from friction are NOT pressure injuries. Pressure injuries arise from pressure in combination with shearing forces.[24] Therefore, understanding the definitions of friction and shear assists in differentiating between these two sources of injury and correctly identifying pressure injuries.

Friction occurs when two surfaces rub together to cause injury, such as the skin sliding across bed linens. Immobility or involuntary muscle movements contribute to the development of friction injuries. Shear occurs when friction prevents the skin from moving with the underlying tissues, which results in compression, stretching, or tearing of the skin. Both friction and shearing injuries are preventable using proper positioning and transfer techniques.[25]

Best Practices for Pressure Injury Prevention – Friction and Shear[4]
• Do not rub or massage areas at risk of developing a pressure injury
• Use silk-like linens
• Support feet when the patient sits upright in a chair
• Place a foam dressing over areas prone to friction and shear for prevention (e.g., heels and sacrum)
• Lift Devices:
o Never drag the patient – use lifting devices
o Remove the lifting device from under patient after use

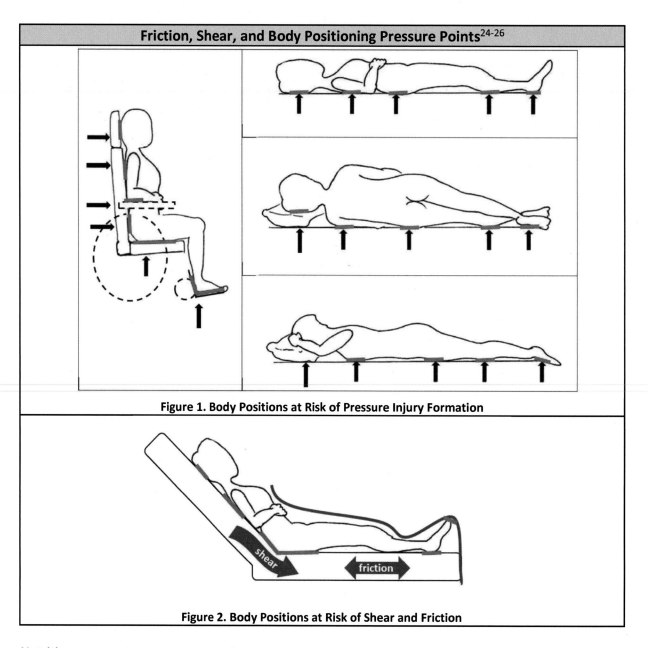

Friction, Shear, and Body Positioning Pressure Points[24-26]

Figure 1. Body Positions at Risk of Pressure Injury Formation

Figure 2. Body Positions at Risk of Shear and Friction

Nutrition
Adequate nutrition is necessary to maintain skin integrity and to heal existing pressure injuries. Nutrition is an extensive topic. See *Nutrition*, page 97, for greater detail in the management of nutritional needs of the palliative patient.

Localized Wound Care
Providing localized wound care is essential in managing the distressing symptoms associated with pressure injuries. After assessing and staging the pressure injury, initiate wound care. Follow appropriate wound care orders that promote a moist wound bed while minimizing pain, controlling odor, preventing infection, and offering a long wear time. Do not debride dry, stable eschar, especially of the heel. Instead, keep the eschar dry by painting the perimeter of the wound with povidone-iodine daily. Use the following algorithms and treatment grids to assist in selecting an appropriate dressing.

WOUND TREATMENT GRID: Pressure Injuries Stage 1 & 2 [4,27-33]

Wound Need	Intervention	Comments
Cleanse	• **Clean wound:** pour normal saline or wound cleanser • **Infection:** irrigate with wound cleanser or antiseptic*	• Irrigate with 4-15 psi: piston syringe (4.2 psi), squeeze bottle+irrigation cap (4.5 psi), or 35 mL syringe+18 gauge needle (8 psi)
Debridement	• Necrotic tissue should not be present in a Stage 1 or 2 pressure injury	• Review staging if slough/eschar are present
Exudate	Stage 1 (select based on contributing factors): • **Moisture:** barrier cream, liquid barrier film • **Pressure:** foam • **Shear:** hydrocolloid, transparent film, foam Stage 2 (select based on exudate level): • **None/Minimal Exudate:** transparent film, hydrocolloid, PMD* • **Moderate Exudate:** foam, calcium alginate, PMD* • **Heavy Exudate:** PMD*, GFD* (Hydrofiber®)	• Consider using barrier ointment/cream if area is difficult to apply dressing • Protect periwound: apply skin barrier film or barrier cream/ointment • Hydrocolloid and transparent film contraindicated in infection • PMDs* can be used on all exudate levels – moisten with saline if wound bed is dry
Infection	• **None/Minimal Exudate:** hydrogel with silver, honey • **Moderate Exudate:** silver alginate, honey alginate, silver foam • **Heavy Exudate:** GFD* (Hydrofiber®) with silver, cadexomer iodine, GV/MB PU foam*	May treat infection empirically: • MRSA: cadexomer iodine, mupirocin*, silver • *Pseudomonas*: cadexomer iodine, acetic acid • VRE: GV/MB PU foam*, silver • MSSA: cadexomer iodine, chlorhexidine, GV/MB PU foam*, mupirocin*, silver
Malodor	• **Cleansers*:** hypochlorous acid (Vashe®), sodium hypochlorite (Dakin's® 0.125%), acetic acid (0.25-0.5%) • **Dressings:** cadexomer iodine, honey, charcoal, silver, metronidazole (Flagyl®) to wound bed, essential oils (wintergreen or lavender) on dressing • **Environmental strategies:** kitty litter, vanilla extract, coffee grounds, dryer sheets placed in room	• Rule out infection • Wound cleansing aids odor control. • Change dressing more often to manage odor (e.g., hydrocolloid every 24-48 hours). • Hydrocolloid dressings tend to create odor (doesn't mean infection is present)
Dead Space	N/A	N/A
Pruritus	• Not usually associated with wound, assess surrounding skin; consider wound care product in use	• Evaluate for contact dermatitis, hypersensitivity, or yeast dermatitis
Bleeding	• **Dressing strategies:** calcium alginate (silver alginate is not hemostatic), non-adherent dressing, or coagulants (gelatin sponge, thrombin) • **Topical/local strategies:** sclerosing agent (silver nitrate), antifibrinolytic agent (tranexamic acid), astringents (alum solution, sucralfate), vasoconstrictive agents [topical oxymetazoline (Afrin®), topical epinephrine]	• Atraumatic removal of dressings – irrigate with normal saline to remove dressings. • Ask: Is the wound infected? Is patient on warfarin? Is transfusion appropriate? • Consider checking: platelet count, PT/INR, vitamin K deficiency • Use topical vasoconstrictors only when bleeding is minimal, oozing, or seeping
Support Surface	• Pressure-redistributing cushion for wheelchair • Select a support surface using table on page 39	• Float heels – support surfaces are NOT used to prevent pressure injuries to heels
Pain	**Nonpharmacological Interventions:** • **Procedural:** moisture-balanced, non-adherent, long-wear dressings; warm saline irrigation to remove dressings; time-outs; patient participation • **Complementary therapies:** music, relaxation, aromatherapy, visualization, meditation **Pharmacological Interventions:** • **Topical/local:** 2% lidocaine; EMLA®; morphine gel • **Systemic:** scheduled and pre-procedural opioid; tricyclic antidepressant; anticonvulsant	• Rule out infection or wound deterioration • Consider placing: hydrocolloid, foam, calcium alginate, PMD*, soft silicone, or hydrogel • EMLA® cream is applied to periwound tissue 60 minutes before the procedure • Morphine gel is only applied to open/inflamed wounds and must be compounded by a pharmacist

*Cleansers: Rinse wound bed with normal saline after using antiseptic cleanser to minimize toxic effects   **GFD:** Gelling fiber dressing
PMD: polymeric membrane dressing (PolyMem®)   **GV/MB PU Foam:** gentian violet/methylene blue (Hydrofera Blue®Ready™)
Topical Antibiotics: Use of a topical antibiotic is NOT recommended due to the potential for adverse reactions and antimicrobial resistance

WOUND TREATMENT GRID: Pressure Injuries Stage 3 & 4 [4,27-33]

Wound Need	Intervention	Comments
Cleanse	• **Clean wound:** pour normal saline or wound cleanser • **Infection/necrosis:** irrigate with wound cleanser or antiseptic*	• Irrigate with 4-15 psi: piston syringe (4.2 psi), squeeze bottle+irrigation cap (4.5 psi), or 35 mL syringe+18 gauge needle (8 psi)
Debridement	• **Dry:** hydrocolloid, hydrogel, transparent film • **Moist:** hydrocolloid, calcium alginate, GFD* (Hydrofiber®) • **Infected:** silver alginate, Dakin's® BID, NaCl IG*	• Stable eschar of heels, toes, or fingers should NOT be debrided – if present, paint perimeter with povidone-iodine (Betadine®) daily. • Apply Dakin's® soaked gauze BID for debridement
Exudate	• **None/Minimal Exudate:** hydrogel, PMD* • **Moderate Exudate:** foam, calcium alginate, PMD* • **Heavy Exudate:** PMD*, GFD* (Hydrofiber®), specialty absorptive	• Pain/bleeding: PMD* or contact layer (PMDs* can be used on all exudate levels – moisten with saline if wound bed is dry) • Protect periwound: skin barrier film/barrier cream
Infection	• **None/Minimal Exudate:** hydrogel with silver, honey • **Moderate Exudate:** silver alginate, honey alginate, silver foam • **Heavy Exudate:** GFD* (Hydrofiber®) with silver, cadexomer iodine, GV/MB PU foam*	May treat infection empirically: • MRSA: cadexomer iodine, mupirocin*, silver • Pseudomonas: cadexomer iodine, acetic acid • VRE: GV/MB PU foam*, silver • MSSA: cadexomer iodine, chlorhexidine, GV/MB PU foam*, mupirocin*, silver
Malodor	• **Cleansers*:** hypochlorous acid (Vashe®), sodium hypochlorite (Dakin's® 0.125%), acetic acid • **Dressings:** cadexomer iodine, honey, charcoal, silver, metronidazole (Flagyl®); essential oils • **Environmental strategies:** kitty litter, vanilla extract, coffee grounds, or dryer sheets placed in room	• Rule out infection • Wound cleansing aids odor control. • Change dressing more often to manage odor (e.g., hydrocolloid every 24-48 hours) • Hydrocolloid dressings tend to create odor (doesn't mean infection is present) • Essential oils: wintergreen or lavender on dressing
Dead Space	• **None/Minimal Exudate:** hydrogel, PMD* • **Moderate Exudate:** foam, calcium alginate, PMD* • **Heavy Exudate:** foam, GFD* (Hydrofiber®), PMD*	• Loosely fill any dead space • Products are available in different forms, such as roping to pack tunneling
Pruritus	• Not usually associated with wound, assess surrounding skin, rule out wound care product	• Evaluate for contact dermatitis, hypersensitivity, or yeast dermatitis
Bleeding	• **Dressing strategies:** calcium alginate (silver alginate is not hemostatic), non-adherent dressing, or coagulants (gelatin sponge, thrombin) • **Topical/local strategies:** sclerosing agent (silver nitrate), antifibrinolytic agent (tranexamic acid), astringents (alum solution, sucralfate), vasoconstrictive agents [topical oxymetazoline (Afrin®), topical epinephrine]	• Atraumatic removal of dressings – irrigate with normal saline to remove dressings. • Ask: Is the wound infected? Is patient on warfarin? Is transfusion appropriate? • Consider checking: platelet count, PT/INR, vitamin K deficiency • Use topical vasoconstrictors only when bleeding is minimal, oozing, or seeping
Support Surface	• Pressure-redistributing cushion for wheelchair • Select a support surface using table on page 39	• Float heels – support surfaces are not used to prevent pressure injuries to heels
Pain	**Nonpharmacological Interventions:** • **Procedural:** moisture-balanced, non-adherent, long-wear dressings; warm saline irrigation to remove dressings; time-outs; patient participation • **Complementary therapies:** music, relaxation, aromatherapy, visualization, meditation **Pharmacological Interventions:** • **Topical/local:** 2% lidocaine; EMLA®, morphine gel • **Systemic:** scheduled and pre-procedural opioid; tricyclic antidepressant; anticonvulsant	• Rule out infection or wound deterioration • Consider placing: hydrocolloid, foam, calcium alginate, PMD*, soft silicone, or hydrogel • EMLA® cream is applied to periwound tissue 60 minutes before the procedure • Morphine gel is only applied to open/inflamed wounds and must be compounded by a pharmacist

*Cleansers: Rinse wound bed with normal saline after using antiseptic cleanser to minimize toxic effects **GFD:** Gelling fiber dressing
PMD: polymeric membrane dressing (PolyMem®) **GV/MB PU Foam:** gentian violet/methylene blue (Hydrofera Blue®Ready™)
NaCl IG: Sodium chloride impregnated gauze (Mesalt®)
Topical Antibiotics: Use a of topical antibiotic is NOT recommended due to the potential for adverse reactions and antimicrobial resistance

Pressure Injury Staging Tool

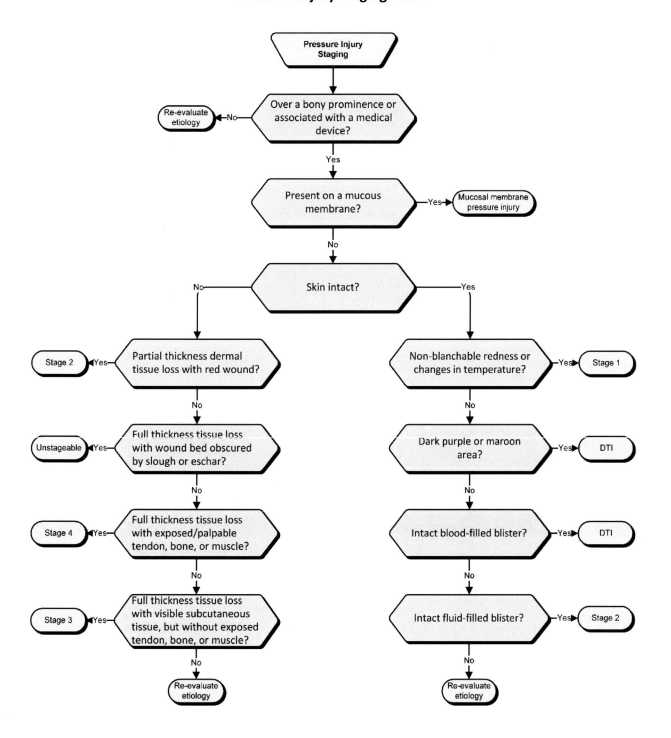

DTI: deep tissue injury

Pressure Injury Management Overview

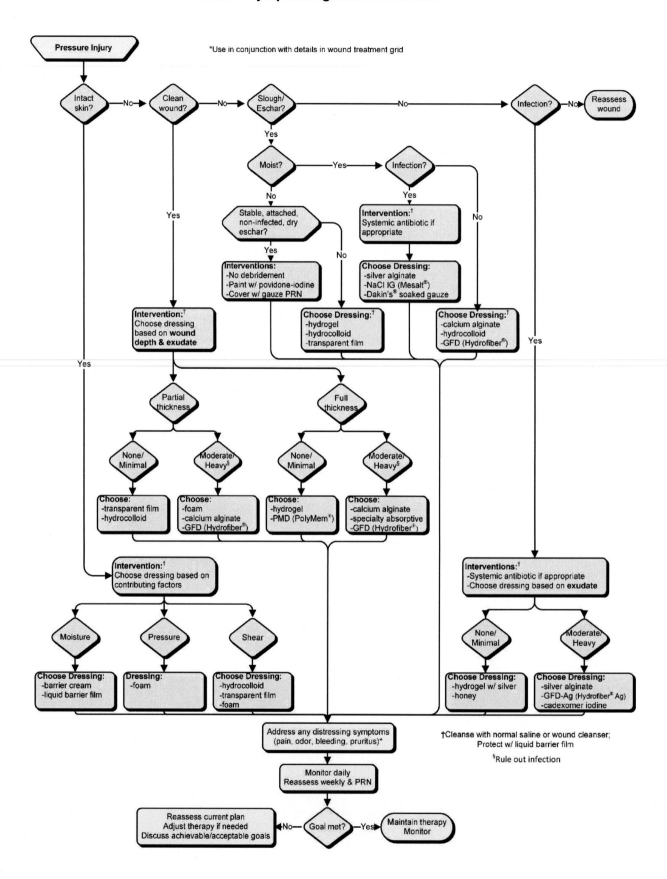

*Use in conjunction with details in wound treatment grid

Pressure Injury

Intact skin? —No→ **Clean wound?** —No→ **Slough/ Eschar?** —No→ **Infection?** —No→ **Reassess wound**

Moist? —Yes→ **Infection?**

No: Stable, attached, non-infected, dry eschar?

Infection? Yes: **Intervention:†** Systemic antibiotic if appropriate

No

Stable, attached, non-infected, dry eschar? **Yes**: **Interventions:** -No debridement -Paint w/ povidone-iodine -Cover w/ gauze PRN

No: **Choose Dressing:†** -hydrogel -hydrocolloid -transparent film

Choose Dressing: -silver alginate -NaCl IG (Mesalt®) -Dakin's® soaked gauze

Choose Dressing:† -calcium alginate -hydrocolloid -GFD (Hydrofiber®)

Clean wound? Yes: **Intervention:†** Choose dressing based on **wound depth & exudate**

Intact skin? Yes

Partial thickness

None/ Minimal → **Choose:** -transparent film -hydrocolloid

Moderate/ Heavy§ → **Choose:** -foam -calcium alginate -GFD (Hydrofiber®)

Full thickness

None/ Minimal → **Choose:** -hydrogel -PMD (PolyMem*)

Moderate/ Heavy§ → **Choose:** -calcium alginate -specialty absorptive -GFD (Hydrofiber®)

Intervention:† Choose dressing based on contributing factors

Moisture → **Choose Dressing:** -barrier cream -liquid barrier film

Pressure → **Dressing:** -foam

Shear → **Choose Dressing:** -hydrocolloid -transparent film -foam

Infection? Yes: **Interventions:†** -Systemic antibiotic if appropriate -Choose dressing based on **exudate**

None/ Minimal → **Choose Dressing:** -hydrogel w/ silver -honey

Moderate/ Heavy → **Choose Dressing:** -silver alginate -GFD-Ag (Hydrofiber® Ag) -cadexomer iodine

Address any distressing symptoms (pain, odor, bleeding, pruritus)*

†Cleanse with normal saline or wound cleanser; Protect w/ liquid barrier film

§Rule out infection

Monitor daily Reassess weekly & PRN

Goal met? —No→ **Reassess current plan Adjust therapy if needed Discuss achievable/acceptable goals**

Goal met? —Yes→ **Maintain therapy Monitor**

Treatment Algorithm for Pressure Injury with Intact Skin (Stage 1)

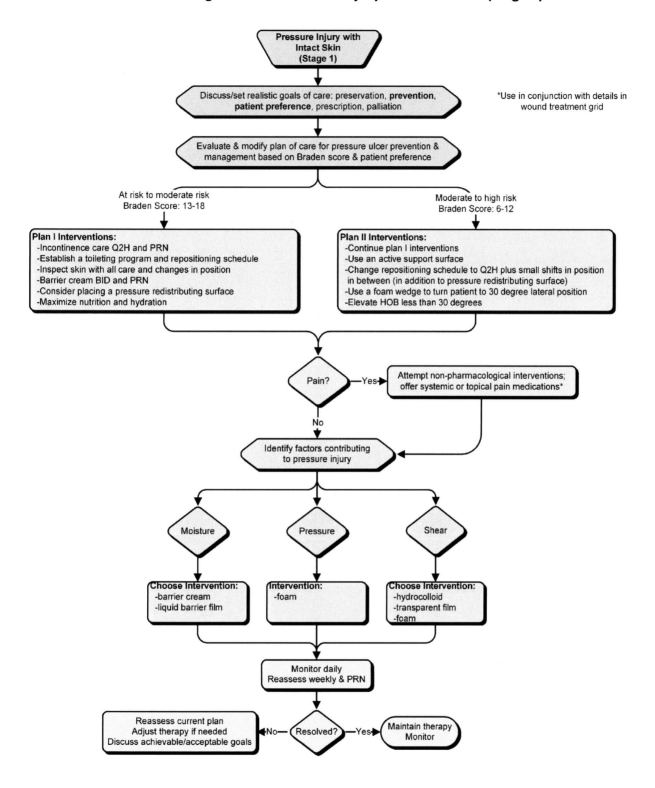

Treatment Algorithm for Pressure Injury with Clean Wound Bed (Stage 2-4)

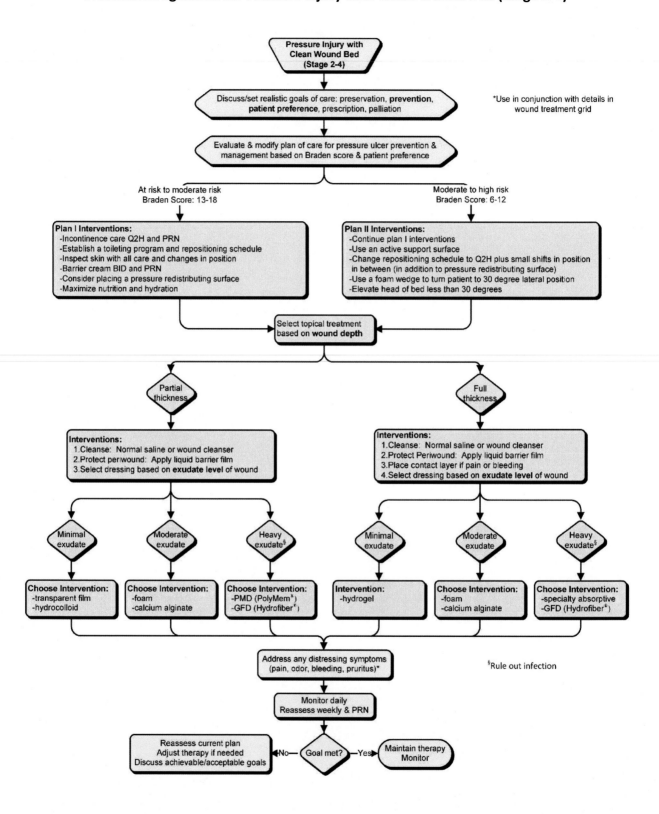

Pressure Injury with Clean Wound Bed (Stage 2-4)

Discuss/set realistic goals of care: preservation, **prevention**, **patient preference**, prescription, palliation

*Use in conjunction with details in wound treatment grid

Evaluate & modify plan of care for pressure ulcer prevention & management based on Braden score & patient preference

At risk to moderate risk
Braden Score: 13-18

Moderate to high risk
Braden Score: 6-12

Plan I Interventions:
-Incontinence care Q2H and PRN
-Establish a toileting program and repositioning schedule
-Inspect skin with all care and changes in position
-Barrier cream BID and PRN
-Consider placing a pressure redistributing surface
-Maximize nutrition and hydration

Plan II Interventions:
-Continue plan I interventions
-Use an active support surface
-Change repositioning schedule to Q2H plus small shifts in position in between (in addition to pressure redistributing surface)
-Use a foam wedge to turn patient to 30 degree lateral position
-Elevate head of bed less than 30 degrees

Select topical treatment based on **wound depth**

Partial thickness

Full thickness

Interventions:
1. Cleanse: Normal saline or wound cleanser
2. Protect periwound: Apply liquid barrier film
3. Select dressing based on **exudate level** of wound

Interventions:
1. Cleanse: Normal saline or wound cleanser
2. Protect Periwound: Apply liquid barrier film
3. Place contact layer if pain or bleeding
4. Select dressing based on **exudate level** of wound

Minimal exudate

Moderate exudate

Heavy exudate§

Minimal exudate

Moderate exudate

Heavy exudate§

Choose Intervention:
-transparent film
-hydrocolloid

Choose Intervention:
-foam
-calcium alginate

Choose Intervention:
-PMD (PolyMem*)
-GFD (Hydrofiber*)

Intervention:
-hydrogel

Choose Intervention:
-foam
-calcium alginate

Choose Intervention:
-specialty absorptive
-GFD (Hydrofiber*)

Address any distressing symptoms (pain, odor, bleeding, pruritus)*

§Rule out infection

Monitor daily
Reassess weekly & PRN

Goal met?

No — Reassess current plan
Adjust therapy if needed
Discuss achievable/acceptable goals

Yes — Maintain therapy Monitor

Treatment Algorithm for Pressure Injury with Slough/Eschar

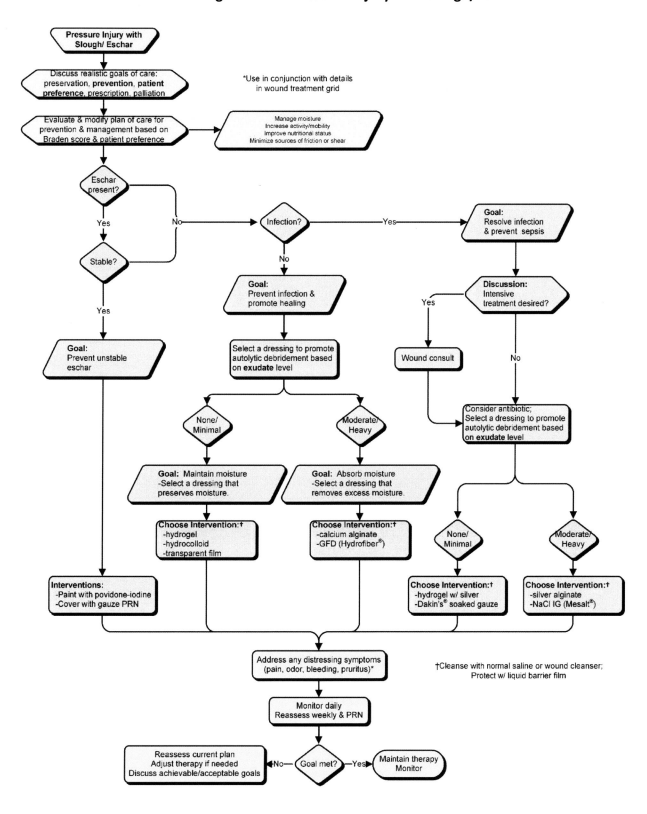

Treatment Algorithm for Pressure Injury with Infection (No Slough)

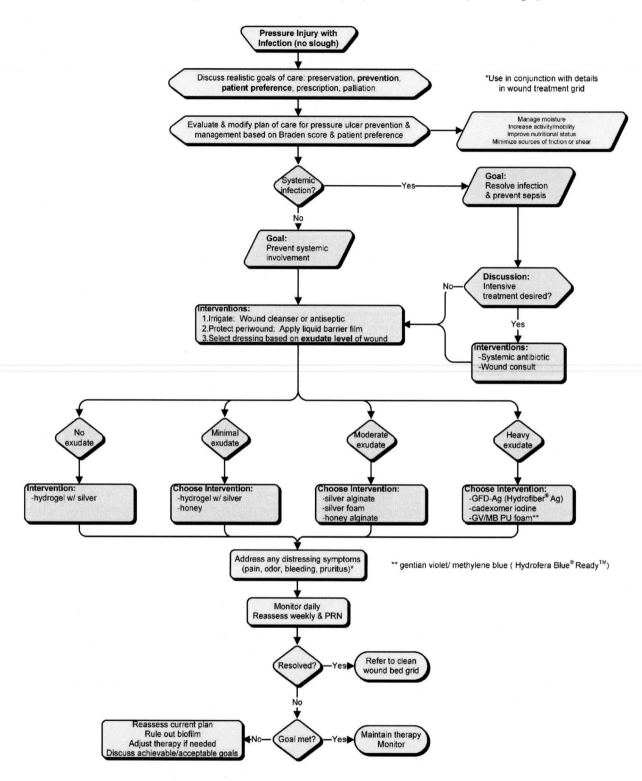

KEY POINTS

- A pressure injury is an area of skin or underlying tissue damage usually associated with a bony prominence or under a medical device.
- Perform a comprehensive assessment to identify patients at risk of, or with, a pressure injury.
- Use a pressure injury risk assessment tool (e.g., The Braden Scale for Predicting Pressure Sore Risk© or The Hunters Hill Marie Curie Centre pressure sore risk assessment tool).
- Stage all pressure injuries using the latest pressure injury staging guidelines from the NPUAP.
- Initiate a plan of care to prevent the development of, or treat, an existing pressure injury.
- Provide localized wound care that promotes a moist wound bed, controls distressing symptoms, and allows for a long wear time.

CASE STUDY

The nurse is visiting a 94-year-old female patient living with her family. The patient has a primary hospice diagnosis of pancreatic cancer. While performing a head to toe assessment, the nurse notes a new pressure injury to the left lateral knee. The nurse performs a comprehensive wound assessment and documents the following:

Stage 3 pressure injury to the left lateral knee measuring 1.4 x 1.7 x 0.2 cm. Wound bed with 60% granulation tissue and 40% slough. Heavy serous drainage. No odor, redness, induration, or edema noted. Wound edges attached but macerated from 3 o'clock to 10 o'clock. No epibole, undermining, or tunneling. Surrounding tissue is warm, dry, and intact. PAINAD pain score 2/10 during wound assessment. Current preventive measures include turning and repositioning frequently (family attempts to turn every 2 to 4 hours), floating heels while in bed, and use of a pressure-redistributing support surface. The patient is incontinent of urine and stool. The family provides incontinence care with each incontinent episode. Barrier cream is applied twice daily and PRN incontinence. Comorbidities include anemia, hypertension, and diabetes mellitus type II. The patient is ordered comfort medications only. Family monitors her finger-stick blood glucose weekly. Her blood glucose level this week was 180 mg/dl. The patient eats approximately 25% of all pureed meals, and the family feeds all meals. Her weight is stable at 114 pounds. She drinks sips of nectar-thickened liquid throughout the day. The patient is bed bound. PPS is 20%. The family wishes to maintain patient's comfort and state that the most distressing symptom is the exudate.

The nurse suggests a polymeric membrane dressing (PolyMem Max®) to both absorb the moderate exudate and promote autolytic debridement. The nurse notifies the physician of her assessment and recommendations. The physician agrees with these recommendations and provides the following wound care orders:

- Irrigate pressure injury to the left lateral knee with normal saline, pat periwound tissue dry. Apply liquid barrier film to periwound tissue. Place a polymeric membrane dressing and secure with paper tape. Change every three days and PRN if soiled.

The nurse reviews the wound care orders with the family, and the family is agreeable to the plan of care. The nurse provides education regarding the application of the dressing and methods for offloading pressure to the area using pillows. The family return-demonstrates the procedures.

References

1. National Pressure Ulcer Advisory Panel (NPUAP). NPUAP pressure injury stages. http://www.npuap.org/resources/educational-and-clinical-resources/npuap-pressure-injury-stages/ Accessed May 2, 2017.
2. National Pressure Ulcer Advisory Panel (NPUAP). The facts about reverse staging in 2000: the NPUAP position statement. http://www.npuap.org/wp-content/uploads/2012/01/Reverse-Staging-Position-Statement%E2%80%A8.pdf Accessed May 3, 2017.
3. Black JM, Edsberg LE, Baharestani MM, et al. Pressure ulcers: avoidable or unavoidable? Results of the national pressure ulcer advisory panel consensus conference. *Ostomy Wound Manage.* 2011;57(2):24-37.
4. National Pressure Ulcer Advisory Panel (NPUAP), European Pressure Ulcer Advisory Panel (EPUAP) and Pan Pacific Pressure Injury Alliance. Prevention and Treatment of Pressure Ulcers: Quick Reference Guide. Emily Haesler (Ed.). Cambridge Media: Osborne Park, Western Australia; 2014.
5. Prevention Plus. Braden Scale for Predicting Pressure Sore Risk http://www.bradenscale.com Accessed May 3, 2017.
6. Chaplin J. Pressure sore risk assessment in palliative care. *J Tissue Viability.* 2000;10(1):27-31.
7. Hampton J, Brosnen C, Hmpley S, et al. Free paper: A comparison of pressure ulcer risk assessment tools in palliative care. *J Tissue Viability.* 2004;14(4):149.
8. Henoch I, Gustafsson M. Pressure ulcers in palliative care: development of a hospice pressure ulcer risk assessment scale. *Int J Palliat Nurs.* 2003;9(11):474-484.
9. National Pressure Ulcer Advisory Panel (NPUAP). Pressure injury prevention points. http://www.npuap.org/resources/educational-and-clinical-resources/pressure-injury-prevention-points/ Accessed May 3, 2017.
10. Wayne G. Impaired tissue integrity. September 13, 2016 https://nurseslabs.com/impaired-tissue-integrity/ Accessed October 12, 2017.
11. Alvarez OM, Kalinski C, Nusbaum J, Hernandez L, et al. Incorporating wound healing strategies to improve palliation (symptom management) in patients with chronic wounds. *J Palliat Med.* 2007;10(5):1161-1189.
12. Hess CT. Managing tissue loads. *Adv Skin Wound Care.* 2008;21(3):144.
13. Spahn J. Support surfaces: science and practice. Presented at First Annual Palliative Wound Care Conference. Hope of Healing Foundation. Cincinnati, Ohio; May 13-14, 2010.
14. National Pressure Ulcer Advisory Panel (NPUAP). Support surface standards initiative (S3I): terms and definitions related to support surfaces. January 29, 2007 http://www.npuap.org/wp-content/uploads/2012/03/NPUAP_S3I_TD.pdf Accessed August 7, 2017.
15. McNichol L, Watts C, Mackey D, et al. Identifying the right surface for the right patient at the right time: generation and content validation of an algorithm for support surface selection. *J Wound Ostomy Continence Nurs.* 2015;42(1):19-37.
16. Wound, Ostomy, and Continence Nurses Society. An evidence- and consensus-based support surface algorithm. http://algorithm.wocn.org/#preventive-braden-subscale-scores Accessed May 4, 2017.
17. Norton L, Coutts P, Sibbald RG. Beds: practical pressure management for surfaces/mattresses. *Adv Skin Wound Care.* 2011;*24*(7):324–332.
18. Registered Nurses' Association of Ontario (RNAO). *Assessment and management of pressure injuries for the interprofessional team.* 3rd ed. Toronto, ON: RNAO; 2016. http://rnao.ca/sites/rnao-ca/files/PI_BPG_FINAL_WEB_June_10_2016.pdf Accessed April 25, 2018.
19. Bryant RA. Types of skin damage and differential diagnosis. In Bryant RA, Nix DP, eds. *Acute & Chronic Wounds: Current Management Concepts.* 4th ed. St Louis, MO:Elsevier/Mosby;2012: 83-107.
20. WoundPedia.com. WoundPedia: evidence informed practice: Ostomy/Continence/Skin Care. http://www.woundpedia.com/ Accessed April 23, 2018.
21. Pieper B. Pressure ulcers: impact, etiology, and classification. In Bryant RA, Nix DP, eds. *Acute & Chronic Wounds: Current Management Concepts.* 4th ed. St Louis, MO:Elsevier/Mosby;2012: 123-136.
22. Ratliff CR. WOCN's evidence-based pressure ulcer guidelines. *Adv Skin Wound Care.* 2005;18(4):204-208.
23. Institute for Clinical Systems Improvement (ICSI). *Health Care Protocol: Skin safety protocol: risk assessment and prevention of pressure ulcers.* March 2007. http://www.cicsp.org/wp-content/uploads/2015/05/Protocolo_para_la_evaluacion_del_riesgo_y_prevencion_de_UPP_En_ingles.pdf Accessed April 23, 2018
24. Antokal S, Brienza D, Bryan N, et al. Friction induced skin injuries – are they pressure ulcers? A National Pressure Ulcer Advisory Panel white paper. November 20, 2012 https://www.npuap.org/wp-content/uploads/2012/01/NPUAP-Friction-White-Paper.pdf. Accessed May 17, 2017.

25. Agency for Health Care Policy and Research (AHCPR). *Pressure ulcers in adults: prediction and prevention.* AHCPR Clinical Practice Guideline no.3; AHCPR-92-0047[archived]. Rockville, MD: AHCPR; 1992. https://www.ncbi.nlm.nih.gov/books/NBK63915/ Accessed April 23, 2018.
26. Agrawal K, Chauhan N. Pressure ulcers: back to basics. Indian J Plast Surg 2012;45(2):244-254
27. Ramundo J. Wound debridement. In Bryant RA, Nix DP, eds. *Acute & Chronic Wounds: Current Management Concepts.* 4th ed. St Louis, MO:Elsevier/Mosby;2012: 279-288.
28. Sibbald RG, Krasner DL, Lutz J. SCALE: Skin changes at life's end: final consensus statement: October 1, 2009. *Adv Skin Wound Care.* 2010;23(5):225-236.
29. Rolstad BS, Bryant RA, Nix DP. Topical management. In Bryant RA, Nix DP, eds. *Acute & Chronic Wounds: Current Management Concepts.* 4th ed. St Louis, MO:Elsevier/Mosby;2012: 289-306.
30. Hopf HW, Shapshak D, Junkins S. Managing wound pain. In Bryant RA, Nix DP, eds. *Acute & Chronic Wounds: Current Management Concepts.* 4th ed. St Louis, MO:Elsevier/Mosby;2012:380-387.
31. Tran QNH, Fancher T. Achieving analgesia for painful ulcers using topically applied morphine gel. *J Support Oncol.* 2007;5(6):289-293.
32. Popescu A, Sal Salcido R. Wound pain: a challenge for the patient and the wound care specialist. *Adv Skin Wound Care.* 2004;17(1):14-20.
33. So-Shn Mak S, Lee MY, Cheung JSS, Choi KC, Chung TK, Wong TW, Lam KY, Lee DT. Pressurised irrigation versus swabbing method in cleansing wounds healed by secondary intention: a randomized controlled trial with cost-effectiveness analysis. *Int J Nurs Stud.* 2015;52:88-101.

KENNEDY TERMINAL ULCERS

GOALS

Within the confines of the patient's prognosis and in alignment with the wishes of the patient and family:

- Assist the patient and family in developing realistic goals of care
- Provide localized wound care to relieve distressing symptoms and promote quality of life

DEFINITIONS

A **Kennedy Terminal Ulcer (KTU)** is an *unavoidable* pressure injury associated with the dying process. It is theorized that as a person begins the dying process, the body enters multi-organ failure and shunts blood from the skin to other vital organs resulting in skin intolerance to any amount of pressure.[1-3] KTUs develop despite the use of pressure-relieving strategies.

ASSESSMENT

A comprehensive wound assessment demonstrates an irregularly shaped blister, abrasion, or intact skin that is red or purple. Despite adequate care, a KTU will rapidly deteriorate to what appears to be a stage 2, 3, or 4 pressure injury. KTUs are typically in the shape of a pear, butterfly or horseshoe with irregular edges. Color can quickly change from red to yellow to black. Although usually seen on the sacrum or coccyx, KTUs can be found over any bony prominence.[1,2]

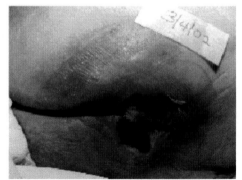

Figure 1. Example of Kennedy Terminal Ulcer[1]

Table 1. Determining Pressure Injury versus Kennedy Terminal Ulcers[1,2,4]	
Pressure Injury	**Kennedy Terminal Ulcer**
• Slow, progressive onset unless adequate prevention & pressure offloading in place • Redness, with firm or boggy consistency • Circular shape, similar to bony prominence below • Potential to prevent progression in most patients • Treat based on current wound conditions	• Rapid onset; interventions do not slow progression • Yellow, brown, purplish-black, with firm consistency • Pear or butterfly shaped, often over buttocks • Poor prognosis; skin failure; unavoidable • Associated with dying process; impending death • Treat based on current wound conditions

PLAN OF CARE

A plan of care for the prevention of a KTU is identical to the prevention of pressure injuries; however, if a KTU develops, the treatment plan of care should focus on the implementation of palliative measures because these wounds will not heal. Table 2 reviews potential care plans for KTUs.[3]

Table 2. Care Plans for Kennedy Terminal Ulcers[3]		
Nursing Diagnosis	**Related Factors**	**Interventions**
Risk for Impaired Skin Integrity • Patient has the potential for an alteration in skin integrity **Impaired Skin Integrity** • Partial thickness tissue loss **Impaired Tissue Integrity** • Full thickness tissue loss	• Terminal phase of an advanced disease process • Inadequate nutrition • Altered sensation or circulation • Immobility • Moisture • Medications	• Assess skin, note areas of discoloration, texture, or temperature and any existing skin alterations • Turn and reposition (state frequency) • Pressure-redistributing surface • Assist with bed mobility and transfers • Maintain skin clean and dry • Incontinence care • Preventive dressings to bony prominences • Maximize nutritional status • Increase activity or mobility, if able • Assess skin alteration and determine etiology • Localized wound care to relieve distressing symptoms, monitor daily

INTERVENTIONS

Treatment of a KTU is similar to that of a pressure injury – treat based on the current wound conditions (*see page 30 for dressing selection*); however, assist the patient and caregiver to set realistic expectations for care outcomes. KTUs will not heal and serve as an ominous sign of impending death. Because the focus of wound care is palliation of symptoms, strive to select dressings that have long wear times, minimize pain, and promote quality of life. KTUs will develop and persist despite the implementation of pressure injury prevention strategies. Therefore, the patient and family should be realistic in their expectations. Even with optimal care, these wounds can continue to deteriorate.[4]

KEY POINTS

• Kennedy Terminal Ulcers are unavoidable skin ulcerations due to the dying process.
• Kennedy Terminal Ulcers develop and deteriorate rapidly and may have the shape of a pear, butterfly, or horseshoe.
• Because Kennedy Terminal Ulcers are an ominous warning sign of impending death and will deteriorate despite providing good wound care, treatment should focus on palliation of symptoms.

CASE STUDY

A 90-year-old female patient admitted to hospice two months ago with a primary diagnosis of Alzheimer's disease. The patient lives at home with her daughter who is her primary caregiver. The patient's past medical history includes congestive heart failure and hypertension. She is bed bound and nonverbal. Yesterday, the daughter noticed a new wound to the patient's coccyx. The nurse completed a comprehensive wound assessment and noted the wound to be a deep tissue pressure injury measuring 2.3 x 1.7 cm. Although the skin was intact, it was dark purple. A bordered foam dressing was ordered for prevention. The nurse also provided the daughter with education regarding the need to continue to provide pressure injury prevention strategies, including turning and repositioning, use of a pressure-redistributing surface, and routine incontinence care. Today, the nurse is called to the home because the daughter noted that the wound looked significantly worse. The nurse reassesses the wound and finds the periwound tissue to be black with necrotic tissue in the wound bed. The wound is butterfly shaped and measures 3.1 x 1.9 cm. Heavy serous drainage is present. The daughter is upset because she feels that the wound deterioration is due to inadequate care; however, the nurse suspects that the wound is a Kennedy Terminal Ulcer. The nurse consults with the physician who provides the diagnosis of a Kennedy Terminal Ulcer. The physician orders a gelling fiber dressing secured with bordered foam to be changed every three days and as needed if soiled. The nurse provides the daughter with education regarding the etiology and prognosis of a Kennedy Terminal Ulcer. The daughter is appreciative of the education. The patient passed away two days later.

References
1. Schank JE. Kennedy terminal ulcer: the "ah-ha!" moment and diagnosis. *Ostomy Wound Manage.* 2009;55(9):40-44. *Image courtesy of Joy Schank; used with permission.*
2. Kennedy-Evans K. Understanding the Kennedy terminal ulcer. *Ostomy Wound Manage.* 2009;55(9):6.
3. Wayne G. Impaired tissue integrity. September 13, 2016 https://nurseslabs.com/impaired-tissue-integrity/ Accessed October 12, 2017.
4. Yastrub DJ. Pressure or pathology distinguishing pressure ulcers from the Kennedy terminal ulcer. *J Wound Ostomy Continence Nurs.* 2010;37(3):249-250.

MOISTURE-ASSOCIATED SKIN DAMAGE (MASD)

GOALS

Within the confines of the patient's prognosis and in alignment with the wishes of the patient and family:

- Maintain skin integrity with individualized prevention strategies
- Heal existing areas of moisture-associated skin damage
- Relieve distressing symptoms and promote quality of life

DEFINITIONS

Moisture-associated skin damage (MASD) is a broad term used to describe skin inflammation and breakdown as a result of persistent contact to various sources of moisture, including urine, stool, perspiration, exudate, saliva, or ostomy effluent. The chemical composition of the moisture, exposure to friction, altered skin pH, and invading organisms contribute to the development of moisture-associated skin damage. MASD may present as red and inflamed skin with or without partial thickness tissue loss. Four types of MASD are recognized:[1]

Types of Moisture-Associated Skin Damage

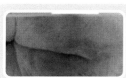

Incontinence-Associated Dermatitis[a]

- Red and inflamed skin with or without partial thickness tissue loss secondary to prolonged or repeated exposure to urine or stool.

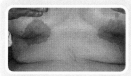

Intertriginous Dermatitis[b]

- Red and inflamed skin with or without partial thickness tissue loss secondary to perspiration and friction.

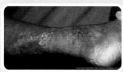

Periwound Moisture-Associated Dermatitis[a]

- Inflammation or maceration of skin secondary to exposure to wound exudate.

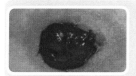

Peristomal Moisture-Associated Dermatitis[a]

- Red and inflamed skin with or without partial thickness tissue loss secondary to exposure to ostomy effluent.

a: image from Medetec Open Access   b: image appears with permission from VisualDx

ASSESSMENT

Completion of a comprehensive skin assessment is the first step to identifying the potential for or any existing areas of moisture-associated skin damage. Assess areas prone to the adverse effects of moisture, including skin folds, perineal area, intergluteal cleft, and periwound or peristomal areas. Differentiate moisture-associated skin damage from pressure injuries by assessing for four clinical features – causative agent, location, depth, and defining characteristics.[1,2] Table 1 provides assessment guidance in differentiating pressure injuries from moisture-associated skin damage.

Table 1. Assessment of Moisture-Associated Skin Damage[1-5]

	Pressure Injuries	Incontinence-Associated Dermatitis	Intertriginous Dermatitis	Periwound Moisture-Associated Dermatitis	Peristomal Moisture-Associated Dermatitis
Definition	• Skin or tissue damage	• Intact, red, and inflamed skin with or without maceration or partial thickness tissue loss (denudation)			
Cause	• Pressure with or without shearing	• Urine • Stool	• Perspiration • Friction • Infection	• Exudate • Skin stripping • Infection	• Stoma effluent (stool or urine) • Infection
Location	• Bony prominences • Under medical devices	• Perineum, groin • Buttocks • Thighs	• Skin folds • Inner thighs • Intergluteal cleft	• Periwound skin	• Peristomal skin
Depth	• Partial or full thickness	• Partial thickness	• Partial thickness	• Partial thickness	• Partial thickness
Defining Features	• Well-defined wound edges • Necrotic tissue, undermining, and tunneling possible	• Diffuse without well-defined wound edges • Necrotic tissue is absent	• Diffuse or linear • Necrotic tissue is absent	• Within 4 cm of wound edge • Necrotic tissue is absent	• Diffuse • Necrotic tissue is absent

PLAN OF CARE

Develop an individualized plan of care to prevent and manage moisture-associated skin damage to guide the actions of all members of the interdisciplinary team. The care plan serves to translate the data gained from completion of the comprehensive skin assessment into a specific plan of action to prevent or treat moisture-associated skin damage. Table 2 reviews potential care plans for MASD.[6]

Table 2. Care Plans for MASD[6]

Nursing Diagnosis	Related Factors	Interventions
Risk for Impaired Skin Integrity • Patient has the potential for an alteration in skin integrity **Impaired Skin Integrity** • Partial thickness tissue loss	• Urine • Stool • Perspiration • Friction • Infection • Exudate • Epidermal stripping • Infection • Ostomy effluent (stool or urine)	• Assess skin, note areas of discoloration, texture, or temperature and any existing skin alterations • Educate patient to adopt healthy skin care routines • Avoid aggravating factors • Incontinence care • Toileting program • Use correctly-fitted ostomy appliance • Use moisture-balanced dressings • Assess skin alteration and determine etiology • Localized wound care, monitor daily • Diversionary devices as needed

INTERVENTIONS

Moisture-associated skin damage causes significant pain and odor for the patient at the end of life. These skin alterations also have the potential to be pruritic.[1] Ultimately, the presence of MASD may lead to a decrease in the quality of life for the palliative patient. Strive to provide preventive care to patients at risk of developing MASD. If MASD develops, management will vary depending upon the etiology of the wound. The following table provides guidance in identifying preventive and curative interventions for MASD, including strategies to control pain, odor, and pruritus.

Table 3. Interventions for the Prevention and Treatment of Moisture-Associated Skin Damage[1-4]				
	Incontinence-Associated Dermatitis (IAD)	Intertriginous Dermatitis (ITD)	Periwound Moisture-Associated Dermatitis	Peristomal Moisture-Associated Dermatitis
Prevention	• Perform incontinence care after each incontinent episode • Address cause of incontinence (e.g., medications, UTI) • Consider timed toileting, use of external catheters, or fecal pouches • Use pH balanced skin cleansers – NOT soap • Moisturize the skin • Apply barrier cream after each incontinent episode (dimethicone or petrolatum-based) • Use briefs only when out of bed	• Keep skin folds clean and dry – pat dry after bathing or allow to air dry • Use a pH balanced cleanser to clean skin folds • Place Tranquility ThinLiner™ Absorbent Sheets in skin folds to retain moisture • Use loose fitting clothes • Choose clothing with natural fibers	• Select a dressing that best matches level of wound exudate • Apply liquid barrier film or barrier cream to periwound skin with each dressing change • Pat periwound edges dry after cleansing wound • Consider using gauze rolls or netting to secure dressings on extremities to prevent tape injury	• Use appropriately sized ostomy barrier, cut to size • Fit the barrier so that only the stoma is exposed • Change pouch as scheduled • Wash peristomal skin with warm water (no soap) and pat dry with every change in pouch
Treatment	*For all types of MASD, initiate preventive measures plus:*			
	• Consider switching to a zinc oxide-based barrier cream if IAD worsens – Do NOT scrub off zinc • Address microclimate – consider mattress, linens, incontinence pads • Domeboro® soaks • Treat fungal or bacterial infection if indicated	• Place InterDry® with antimicrobial silver in affected skin fold, change every 5 days • Treat fungal rash with antifungals • If ITD remains, use 1% hydrocortisone cream/ointment twice daily for 3-5 days	• Use a product with a higher absorptive capacity to manage exudate • Evaluate wound for symptoms of infection and treat accordingly	• Use fillers to prevent leakage • Crusting (denuded skin): 1. Apply light dusting of stomahesive powder; remove any excess. 2. Pat area with liquid barrier film; allow to dry. Repeat layers x 2 • Fungal rash: nystatin powder, change stoma pouch with each application
Management of Associated Symptoms	*Pain, odor, and pruritus are common symptoms of MASD. To manage these symptoms:* • Treat underlying cause • Premedicate before incontinence care or application of treatment • Apply creams to an abdominal pad or gauze and place on impaired skin • Use diversion devices			
Note: Brand names provided as examples of common products; no brand endorsement implied				

KEY POINTS

- Moisture-associated skin damage is a broad term used to describe skin inflammation and breakdown as a result of persistent contact to various sources of moisture, including urine, stool, perspiration, exudate, saliva, or ostomy effluent.

- Moisture-associated skin damage is classified into four categories: incontinence-associated dermatitis, intertriginous dermatitis, periwound moisture-associated dermatitis, and peristomal moisture-associated dermatitis.

- Prevent moisture-associated skin damage by following basic patient care strategies, including patient education, healthy skin care routines, avoidance of aggravating factors, incontinence care, use of moisture-balanced dressings, and use of a correctly-fitted ostomy appliance.

- Treatment will vary depending upon the etiology of the wound.

CASE STUDY

A 69-year-old male patient admitted to hospice one week ago with a primary diagnosis of congestive heart failure. The patient lives in a skilled nursing facility. The patient's past medical history is positive for lymphedema of the lower extremities and hypertension. He is bed bound but alert and oriented. While completing a full body assessment, the facility nurse notes redness to the skin folds of bilateral lower extremities. The nurse consults the hospice who recommends InterDry® with antimicrobial silver be placed in the skin folds and changed every five days. After resolution of the redness, the hospice recommends switching to Tranquility ThinLiner™ Absorbent Sheets in skin folds to retain moisture and prevent further instances of intertriginous dermatitis.

References

1. Gray M, Black JM, Baharestani MM, et al. Moisture-associated skin damage overview and pathophysiology. *J Wound Ostomy Continence Nurs.* 2011;38(3):233-241.
2. Idensohn T. Differential assessment: pressure ulcers versus incontinence-associated dermatitis versus intertriginous dermatitis. *Wound Healing Southern Africa.* 2015;8(1):31-33.
3. Junkin J. Incontinence-associated dermatitis intervention tool (IADIT). 2008. http://ltctoolkit.rnao.ca/sites/default/files/resources/continence/Continence_EducationResources/IADIT.pdf Accessed May 9, 2017.
4. Kennedy-Evans K, Smith D, Viggiano B, et al. Multisite feasibility study using a new textile with silver for management of skin conditions located in skin folds: 1431. *J Wound Ostomy Continence Nurs.* 2007;34(3S):S68.
5. National Pressure Ulcer Advisory Panel (NPUAP). NPUAP Pressure Injury Stages. http://www.npuap.org/resources/educational-and-clinical-resources/npuap-pressure-injury-stages/ Accessed May 2, 2017.
6. Vera M. Four dermatitis nursing care plans. January 25, 2012 https://nurseslabs.com/dermatitis-nursing-care-plans/ Accessed October 13, 2017.

LOWER EXTREMITY ULCERS

Lower extremity ulceration is a prevalent and debilitating condition that reflects an advanced disease process. The three primary types of lower extremity ulcerations are venous ulcers, arterial ulcers, and diabetic foot ulcers. Presence of a lower extremity ulcer is associated with pain and infection for individuals at the end of life. Management of wound symptoms is critical to improving quality of life; however, improper management of a lower extremity ulcer can result in rapid deterioration of the wound, increased suffering for the patient, and increased caregiver burden. Understanding the etiology of each type of lower extremity ulcer will assist in recognizing the distinguishing characteristics of these ulcers. The underlying disease process and resulting wound characteristics will guide treatment for the palliative care patient.

Reference
1. Spentzouris G, Labropoulos N. The evaluation of lower-extremity ulcers. *Semin Intervent Radiol.* 2009;26(40):286-295.

ARTERIAL ULCERS

GOALS

Within the confines of the patient's prognosis and in alignment with the wishes of the patient and family:

- Maintain skin integrity with individualized prevention strategies
- Preserve existing areas of arterial ulcers to prevent infection
- Relieve distressing symptoms and promote quality of life

DEFINITIONS

Lower extremity arterial disease (LEAD) is caused by reduced arterial blood flow primarily due to atherosclerosis. The reduction in arterial blood supply causes hypoxia and subsequent tissue damage and necrosis, which is evident by the appearance of an **arterial ulcer**. Arterial ulcers are also the result of localized injury in the presence of advanced lower extremity arterial disease. **Intermittent claudication**, defined as pain with ambulation that resolves with rest, is a classic symptom of this disease.[1]

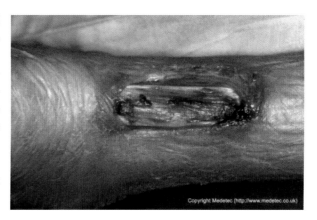

Figure 1. Lower Extremity Arterial Disease

ASSESSMENT

Arterial ulcers present as "punched out" lesions on the lower legs, feet, or toes. Necrotic tissue is usually present. If visualized, the wound bed is pale with little to no exudate. Dorsalis pedis and posterior tibial pulses can be decreased or absent. The skin may be thin, shiny, and dry – usually hairless and may be cool to touch, appear pale, or cyanotic. The toenails may be thickened or lost. Pain increases as the severity of the disease worsens and is usually severe. Elevating the extremity can cause the pain to worsen; dangling the lower extremities over the side of the bed or sitting in a chair may relieve the pain.[1]

Assess the extent of lower extremity arterial disease using the Ankle Brachial Index (ABI), which gauges arterial disease from mild to severe. The ABI is equal to the ankle systolic pressure divided by the brachial systolic pressure. An index of 1 to 1.1 is normal, while an index of 0.90 or less indicates arterial disease. An index of 0.40 or less is severe, and loss of limb is possible (critical limb ischemia). The ABI is a guide for treatment but should not supersede assessment. Critical limb ischemia is possible even with a normal ABI.[1] If an arterial ulcer is present, an ABI less than 0.7 indicates that the wound will likely not heal without revascularization.[2]

Certain disease states, such as diabetes, renal failure, or arthritis, cause elevation of the ABI due to calcification of the arteries rendering the arteries noncompressible. If this is the case, the ABI is greater than 1.30. Obtain toe pressures for an ABI greater than 1.30 to determine a toe brachial index (TBI). A TBI of less than 0.64 indicates arterial disease. Systolic toe pressures less than 30 mmHg or less than 50 mmHg in a diabetic patient suggests severe ischemia, and loss of limb is possible (critical limb ischemia). Complete assessment of perfusion status also includes evaluation of temperature, color, sensation, capillary refill (abnormal result is greater than 3 seconds) and transcutaneous oxygen (hypoxia is less than 40 mmHg).[3]

PLAN OF CARE

Develop an individualized plan of care to prevent or treat arterial ulcers to guide the actions of all members of the interdisciplinary team. The care plan serves to translate the data gained from the comprehensive assessment into a specific plan of action to prevent or manage arterial ulcers. Table 1 includes potential care plan information for arterial ulcers.[1,4,5]

Table 1. Plan of Care for Arterial Ulcers		
Nursing Diagnosis	**Related Factors**	**Interventions**
Risk for Impaired Skin Integrity • Potential for an alteration in skin integrity **Impaired Skin Integrity** • Partial thickness skin alteration **Impaired Tissue Integrity** • Full thickness tissue loss	• Reduced/inadequate tissue perfusion • Inadequate nutrition • Pressure • Cardiovascular disease • Vascular procedures • Sickle cell anemia • Smoking • Knowledge deficit • Trauma	• Assess skin, note discoloration, texture, or temperature and any existing skin alterations • Relieve pain • Revascularization surgery • Maintain adequate nutrition and hydration • Maintain legs in a neutral or dependent position • Walking 3 times/week for 30 - 45 minutes • Protect lower extremities from trauma • Monitor lower extremities and feet daily • Assess skin alteration and determine etiology, reassess regularly, monitor daily • Localized wound care, prevent/treat infection

INTERVENTIONS

Lower extremity arterial disease is progressive. Strive to reduce disease progression by addressing modifiable risk factors, such as smoking cessation and controlling hypertension, hyperlipidemia, and diabetes; however, as the disease progresses, surgical revascularization may be necessary to correct the underlying ischemia. In the palliative care patient, these treatment options may not be useful, practical, or desired. Therefore, focus on the prevention of arterial ulcers. The primary method of preventing the development of arterial ulcers is protecting the lower extremities and feet from trauma. Encourage the patient to wear good fitting shoes, offload pressure to heels, refrain from walking barefoot, and avoid heating pads. In addition to protecting the lower extremities from trauma, recommend discontinuation of vasoconstrictive medications, such as non-selective beta blockers, if able, and limit exposure to restrictive clothing, caffeine, and cold temperatures.[1,4]

Localized Wound Care
Palliative management of the arterial ulcer is unique. Traditionally, the principles of moist wound healing and wound bed preparation assist in managing the symptoms of the wound; however, without revascularization and in the presence of inadequate perfusion, the wound will likely not heal. The risk of developing an infection is high and can pose a threat to life, limb, and quality of life; only use moist wound healing when perfusion to the extremity is adequate or the limb is revascularized and close monitoring of the wound is possible. In the presence of inadequate perfusion, strive for a dry wound bed.[2-4,6]

Do not debride arterial ulcers despite presence of slough and eschar because of the potential for further ischemia and increase in wound size. Keep dry eschar dry by painting the perimeter of the wound with povidone-iodine. If exudate is present, cadexomer iodine applied to the perimeter of the wound bed daily will assist in drying the wound, preventing wet gangrene and infection. Apply dry gauze or a clean sock to protect the area if needed. Infection is common in arterial ulcers and can cause rapid decline in the wound. If an infection is suspected, systemic antibiotics are necessary in addition to topical antimicrobials.[2-4,6]

Left untreated, peripheral arterial disease can lead to gangrene. Dry gangrene is the result of a gradual loss of blood flow to the tissues causing the tissues to die and turn black. A unique characteristic of dry gangrene is the line of demarcation between healthy tissue and dead tissue.[1] Treat dry gangrene by painting the perimeter of the affected area with povidone-iodine daily and leaving open to air. Dry gangrene can deteriorate and become wet gangrene. Use the following algorithms and treatment grids to assist in selecting an appropriate dressing.

Table 2. Best Practices for the Management of Arterial Ulcers[2,3]	
Debridement	• Do not debride dry, stable eschar unless perfusion is adequate and healing is possible • If infected, consider surgical debridement with revascularization • Trial autolytic or enzymatic debridement only if perfusion status is known and if the wound can be closely monitored for infection/deterioration

Dressing Selection	• Allow perfusion status to guide wound treatment selection:
	  • Dry wound healing: inadequate perfusion, revascularization not possible or desired, palliative care
	  • Moist wound healing: adequate perfusion, revascularization achieved, close monitoring is possible
	• Dry, non-infected wounds with stable necrotic tissue: maintain dry wound bed, no debridement
	• Infected wound with any necrotic tissue: Refer for surgical consult, culture-guided systemic antibiotics
	• Avoid occlusive dressings; select a dressing the allows for frequent visualization of the wound bed

Infection	• Monitor closely for signs and symptoms of infection • Topical antimicrobials should not be the sole treatment of an infection – systemic antibiotics are needed; antibiotic selection is guided by cultures • Infected wounds with severe ischemia need immediate evaluation and antibiotic therapy

WOUND TREATMENT GRID: Arterial or Ischemic Ulcers[1-4,6-8]

Wound Need	Intervention	Comments
Cleanse	• Normal saline or commercial wound cleanser only if healing is the goal • Povidone-iodine or antimicrobial solution if attempting to dry wound	• Avoid the use of moisture in dry eschar or dry necrosis where the goal is to maintain a dry wound bed
Debridement	• Debridement is NOT recommended unless perfusion status is known • Infection/wet gangrene: surgical consult	• Attempt to dry the wound bed despite the presence of slough or eschar
Exudate	• **Stable eschar**: paint perimeter of wound with povidone-iodine (Betadine®) or an antimicrobial solution (if iodine is contraindicated) daily and leave open to air • **Moist necrosis, slough**: paint moist areas with povidone-iodine (Betadine®) BID or apply cadexomer iodine paste to wound perimeter daily; GFD* (Hydrofiber®) with silver (if iodine is contraindicated) • **Adequate perfusion**: trial of PMD* or GFD* (Hydrofiber®) with silver (moistened with saline for dry wound bed)	• Select a dressing to dry the wound bed – healing is not the goal unless the underlying ischemia can be resolved • Use caution when applying a dressing – ensure it is not too tight • Do NOT use occlusive dressings, can protect with gauze as needed • Use silver for moist wound healing to prevent/treat infection
Infection	• Continue use of topical antimicrobial dressings* • Add culture-guided systemic antibiotic therapy • Consider surgical consult for symptom palliation (e.g., pain) if desired by patient	• Can be difficult to diagnose due to minimal symptoms • Common with arterial ulcers • Keep clean and dry, monitor daily
Malodor	• **Dressing strategies:** cadexomer iodine, charcoal, essential oils (wintergreen or lavender) placed on dressing • **Environmental strategies:** kitty litter, vanilla extract, coffee grounds, or dryer sheets placed in room	• Evaluate for infection or gangrene
Dead Space	• Use products above to loosely fill any dead space	• Dressing materials placed into open wounds to fill dead space.
Pruritus	• Not usually associated with wound, assess surrounding skin.	• Evaluate for contact dermatitis, hypersensitivity, or yeast dermatitis
Bleeding	• **Dressing strategies:** calcium alginate (silver alginate is not hemostatic), non-adherent dressings, coagulants (gelatin sponge, thrombin), atraumatic removal of dressings • **Topical/local strategies:** sclerosing agent (silver nitrate), antifibrinolytic agent (tranexamic acid), astringents (alum solution, sucralfate), vasoconstrictive agents [topical oxymetazoline (Afrin®), topical epinephrine]	• Rare due to poor perfusion • Ask: Is the wound infected? Is patient on warfarin? Is transfusion appropriate? • Consider checking: platelet count, PT/INR, vitamin K deficiency • Use topical vasoconstrictors only when bleeding is minimal, oozing, or seeping
Support Surface	• Place support surface if pressure was causative injury leading to development of arterial ulceration	• What is the causative injury?
Pain	**Nonpharmacological Interventions:** • **Procedural:** time-outs; patient participation; non-adherent dressings; avoid elevation, allow patient to dangle lower extremities • **Complementary therapies:** music, relaxation, aromatherapy, visualization, meditation **Pharmacological Interventions:** • **Systemic:** scheduled and pre-procedural opioid; tricyclic antidepressant; anticonvulsant; antiplatelet agents, such as cilostazol (Pletal®)	• Rule out infection and wound deterioration • Encourage ambulation • Pain is often severe – even at rest • Elevation of extremity may increase pain; dangling legs over side of bed may relieve pain • Cilostazol (Pletal®) is contraindicated in patients with heart failure – any level of severity.

*GFD: Gelling fiber dressing
PMD: polymeric membrane dressing (PolyMem®)
Topical Antibiotics: Use of a topical antibiotic is NOT recommended due to the potential for adverse reactions and antimicrobial resistance

Treatment Algorithm for Arterial Ulcer

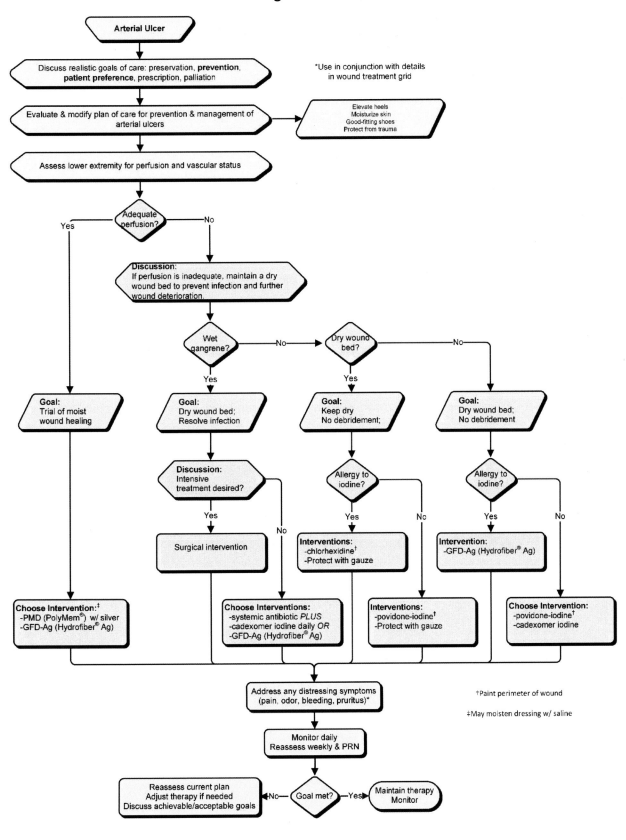

KEY POINTS

- Arterial ulcers result from tissue hypoxia, or localized injury, in the presence of advanced lower extremity arterial disease.
- Prevention of ulcer development is the primary focus for the palliative care population.
- Localized wound care of an arterial ulcer at the end of life requires keeping the wound bed dry.
- Do not attempt debridement of an arterial ulcer unless the perfusion status is known, wound healing is possible, and the ulcer can be closely monitored.

CASE STUDY

The nurse is admitting a 76-year-old male patient to hospice with a primary diagnosis of CVA. While performing a head to toe assessment, the nurse notes an arterial ulcer to the left lateral foot measuring 1.5 x 0.9 cm. The wound bed is 100% dry, stable eschar. No odor, exudate, redness, induration, or edema is noted. The surrounding skin is cool, dry, and intact. The patient's pain is controlled with current oral medications. The family wishes to maintain patient's comfort and currently cares for the wound by washing daily with soap and water and applying a gauze dressing. The nurse educates the family on preventive strategies for arterial ulcers, including protecting the feet and lower extremities from trauma. The nurse suggests discontinuing the daily washes with soap and water because this could result in unstable eschar. Instead, the nurse suggests painting the perimeter of the wound with povidone-iodine daily. The nurse notifies the physician of her assessment and recommendations. The physician agrees with the nurse's assessment and provides the following orders:

- Paint perimeter of arterial ulcer left lateral foot with povidone-iodine daily and protect with a clean sock or dry gauze as needed.

The nurse reviews the wound care orders with the family, and the family is agreeable to the plan of care. The nurse provides education regarding the application of the povidone-iodine and the gauze. The family return-demonstrates the procedures.

References

1. Grey JE, Harding KG, Enoch S. Venous and arterial ulcers. *BMJ*. 2006;332(7537):347-350.
2. Wound Ostomy and Continence Nurses Society. A quick reference guide for lower-extremity wounds: venous, arterial, and neuropathic. April 4, 2013. http://c.ymcdn.com/sites/www.wocn.org/resource/collection/E3050C1A-FBF0-44ED-B28B-C41E24551CCC/A_Quick_Reference_Guide_for_LE_Wounds_(2013).pdf. Accessed July 14, 2017.
3. Bonham P, Flemister B, Droste L, et al. 2014 guideline for management of wounds in patients with lower-extremity arterial disease (LEAD): an executive summary. *J Wound Ostomy Continence Nurs* 2016;43(1):23-31.
4. Takahashi P. Chronic ischemic, venous, and neuropathic ulcers in long-term care. *Ann LTC* 2006;14(7):26-31.
5. Wayne G. Impaired tissue integrity. September 13, 2016 https://nurseslabs.com/impaired-tissue-integrity/ Accessed October 12, 2017.
6. Williams RL. Cadexomer iodine: an effective palliative dressing in chronic critical limb ischemia. *Wounds*. 2009;21(1):15-28
7. Jones V, Grey JE, Harding KG. Wound dressings. *BMJ*. 2006;332(7544):777-780.
8. Popescu A, Sal Salcido R. Wound pain: a challenge for the patient and the wound care specialist. *Adv Skin Wound Care*. 2004;17(1):14-20.

VENOUS ULCERS

GOALS

Within the confines of the patient's prognosis and in alignment with the wishes of the patient and family:

- Maintain skin integrity with individualized prevention strategies
- Preserve existing areas of venous ulcers to prevent infection
- Relieve distressing symptoms and promote quality of life

DEFINITIONS

Lower extremity venous disease (LEVD) is the pooling of venous blood in the lower extremities usually due to incompetent venous valves that are unable to facilitate the return of blood back to the heart. If left untreated, venous ulcerations can develop. Risk factors for the development of venous disease and subsequent ulcerations include a history of varicose veins, leg fracture, deep vein thrombosis, obesity, or a family history of chronic venous insufficiency.[1] In addition to chronic venous insufficiency, medications or other disease processes, such as dysfunction of the heart, liver, or kidneys, can exacerbate venous disease and lead to ulceration.[2]

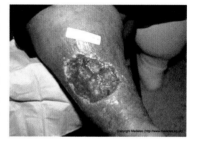

Figure 2. Lower Extremity Venous Disease

ASSESSMENT

Venous ulcers occur on the lower extremities between the ankles and the knees or on the malleoli. An ulcer may present in one area of the lower extremity or circumferentially around the entire limb. These wounds are usually shallow with irregular edges. Exudate level is moderate to heavy due to the associated edema. Granulation tissue or slough is usually present in the wound bed. Venous insufficiency also causes extravasation of erythrocytes leading to deposition of hemosiderin, a protein resulting from breakdown of hemoglobin, in the skin. Hemosiderin staining can be seen in the skin surrounding venous ulceration and appears as hyperpigmentation of the skin above the ankles. Lipodermatosclerosis often ensues. In lipodermatosclerosis, the dermis and subcutaneous tissue become fibrotic. Sweat glands and hair follicles are lost. The skin varies in color from hypopigmented to hyperpigmented. As lipodermatosclerosis progresses, the leg resembles an "inverted champagne bottle." Pain is described as a dull ache or heaviness that is relieved with elevation of the lower extremities.[1-4]

PLAN OF CARE

Develop an individualized plan of care to prevent or treat venous ulcers to guide the actions of all members of the interdisciplinary team. The care plan serves to translate the data gained from completion of the comprehensive assessment into a specific plan of action to prevent or manage venous ulcers. Table 3 includes potential care plans for venous ulcers.[3,5]

Table 3. Plan of Care for Venous Ulcers		
Nursing Diagnosis	**Related Factors**	**Interventions**
Risk for Impaired Skin Integrity • Patient has the potential for an alteration in skin integrity **Impaired Skin Integrity** • Partial thickness tissue loss **Impaired Tissue Integrity** • Full thickness tissue loss	• Inadequate nutrition • History of DVT • History of leg ulcerations • History of trauma • Obesity • Smoking • CHF, renal or liver disease • Impaired mobility • Prior vascular surgery • Knowledge deficit	• Assess skin, note discoloration, texture, or temperature and any existing skin alterations • Assist with bed mobility, transfers, and ambulation • Maintain skin clean and dry, moisturize intact skin • Increase venous return: compression, elevation of lower extremities, ambulation, smoking cessation, and weight loss • Protect from trauma; avoid prolonged standing, crossing legs, and restrictive clothing • Assess skin alteration and determine etiology, reassess regularly, monitor daily • Localized wound care, prevent/treat infection • Relieve pain

INTERVENTIONS

Prevention

Compression is the primary prevention and treatment intervention of lower extremity venous disease and venous ulcers if arterial blood flow is adequate. A multilayer elastic compression system is preferred. Strive for 30-42 mmHg of compression at the ankle.[3] Note that anti-embolism stockings (e.g., TED hose) do not provide adequate compression. Do not use anti-embolism stockings to prevent or treat lower extremity edema. The Unna's boot may be used in the management of venous ulcers. It is an inelastic (rigid) dressing, which consists of gauze impregnated with zinc oxide, calamine, and other ingredients.[1] The Unna's boot does not provide compression, but improves the function of the calf muscle pump. Therefore, the Unna's boot is only appropriate for ambulatory patients.

For the palliative care or hospice patient, compression may or may not be in alignment with their goals of care. Some patients find that compression reduces edema and helps to relieve pain, while others dislike the use of compression devices. Discuss the use of compression, if any, with the patient prior to implementation. If the patient wishes to use compression, selection of the appropriate device is necessary.[6] Factors to consider when selecting a compression method include:[7]

- Consider using a multi-layer system that contains an elastic layer. An elastic component added to two and three component systems might be beneficial.
- Anti-embolism stockings or hose (15-17 mmHg) are *not* designed for therapeutic compression.

- Consider modified, reduced compression bandaging (23-30 mmHg at the ankle) for mixed arterial/venous disease and moderate arterial insufficiency (ABI: 0.5-0.8) for patients with ulcers and edema. Do not apply compression to the lower extremity if the ABI is less than 0.5.
- Consider using intermittent pneumatic compression (IPC) for patients who are immobile or who have not responded to stockings/wraps.

If the patient does not wish to use compression to improve venous return, consider using other methods to improve venous return:[3]

- When sitting, elevate the legs above the heart – attempt to elevate for 30 minutes, four times daily.
- Increase physical activity if able – walking, calf exercises, toe lifts, or ankle exercises.
- Avoid crossing legs, wearing restrictive clothing, or prolonged standing.

Localized Wound Care
Managing the venous ulcer with the use of topical dressings follows the principles of moist wound healing and wound bed preparation. Selection of a wound care product depends on the characteristics of the wound bed.[2] No particular product demonstrates superiority over another in healing a venous leg ulcer.[8] The placement of compression, not topical wound dressings, is primarily responsible for the resolution of these wounds. Therefore, in hospice and palliative care, dressing selection should hinge on what is comfortable for the patient while managing the symptoms of the wound. High levels of exudate are a characteristic of these ulcers. Manage this exudate to prevent maceration of the wound edges and painful deterioration of the wound.[2] Calcium alginate and foam are useful when managing exudate. If the exudate level decreases, switch the dressing to a hydrocolloid.[9]

Infection and Dermatitis
Infection may occur; if systemic antibiotics are needed to manage symptoms, consider recommending an appropriate agent based on culture and sensitivity if in alignment with the goals and wishes of the patient. Venous eczema, also known as stasis dermatitis, is common and is distinct from cellulitis. Venous eczema results in a painful, erythematous extremity that may weep, itch or scale. Treat venous eczema with topical corticosteroids for one to two weeks and emollients (e.g., petrolatum).[1] Because skin with dermatitis is already sensitive, avoid use of topical emollients that contact fragrances, dyes, or perfumes.[10] Use the following algorithms and treatment grids to assist in selecting an appropriate dressing.

WOUND TREATMENT GRID: Venous Ulcers[1-3,7-17]

Wound Need	Intervention	Comments
Cleanse	<ul><li>**Clean wound bed:** normal saline or wound cleanser</li><li>**Infection/necrosis:** irrigate with wound cleanser or antiseptic*</li></ul>	<ul><li>Irrigate with 4-15 psi: piston syringe (4.2 psi), squeeze bottle+irrigation cap (4.5 psi), or 35 mL syringe+18 gauge needle (8 psi)</li></ul>
Debridement	<ul><li>**Dry:** hydrogel, hydrocolloid</li><li>**Moist:** calcium alginate, hydrocolloid, hydroconductive</li><li>**Infected:** cadexomer iodine, GV/MB PU foam*, NaCl IG*</li></ul>	<ul><li>Stable eschar of heels, toes, or fingers should NOT be debrided – paint perimeter with povidone-iodine (Betadine®) daily</li></ul>
Exudate	<ul><li>**None/Minimal Exudate:** hydrogel, hydrocolloid, PMD*</li><li>**Moderate Exudate:** calcium alginate, foam, PMD*</li><li>**Heavy:** GFD* (Hydrofiber®), hydroconductive, PMD*</li></ul>	<ul><li>PMD* – moisten with saline if dry wound bed</li><li>Protect periwound: skin barrier film, barrier cream</li></ul>
Infection	<ul><li>**None/Minimal Exudate:** hydrogel with silver</li><li>**Moderate Exudate:** silver alginate, silver foam</li><li>**Heavy Exudate:** GFD* (Hydrofiber®) with silver, cadexomer iodine, GV/MB PU foam*</li><li>Culture-guided systemic antibiotic if deeper infection</li></ul>	May treat infection empirically:<ul><li>MRSA: cadexomer iodine, mupirocin*, silver</li><li>Pseudomonas: cadexomer iodine, acetic acid</li><li>VRE: GV/MB PU foam*, silver</li><li>MSSA: cadexomer iodine, chlorhexidine, GV/MB PU foam*, mupirocin*, silver</li></ul>
Malodor	<ul><li>**Cleansers*:** hypochlorous acid (Vashe®), sodium hypochlorite (Dakin's® 0.125%), acetic acid (0.25-0.5%)</li><li>**Dressings:** cadexomer iodine, honey, charcoal, silver, metronidazole (Flagyl®), essential oils</li><li>**Environmental strategies:** kitty litter, vanilla extract, coffee grounds, or dryer sheets placed in room</li></ul>	<ul><li>Wound cleansing aids odor control.</li><li>Change dressing more often to manage odor (e.g., hydrocolloid every 24-48 hours).</li><li>Hydrocolloid dressings tend to create odor (doesn't mean infection is present)</li><li>Essential oils: lavender, wintergreen</li></ul>
Dead Space	<ul><li>**None/Minimal Exudate:** hydrogel, PMD*</li><li>**Moderate/Heavy Exudate:** calcium alginate, foam, PMD*, GFD* (Hydrofiber®), hydroconductive</li></ul>	<ul><li>Loosely fill any dead space</li><li>Products are available in different forms, such as roping to pack tunneling</li></ul>
Pruritus	<ul><li>Stasis dermatitis: use emollients (Lubriderm®, Eucerin®, Keri®, Aquaphor® or petrolatum)</li><li>Corticosteroids (topical OTC creams first, burst of oral corticosteroids if severe): Cortaid®, Kenalog®</li></ul>	<ul><li>Stasis dermatitis and pruritus are common. Stasis dermatitis may mimic cellulitis. Avoid antibiotics unless bacterial infection is present.</li></ul>
Bleeding	<ul><li>**Dressing strategies:** calcium alginate (silver alginate is not hemostatic), non-adherent dressing (e.g., contact layer), or coagulants (gelatin sponge, thrombin)</li><li>**Topical/local strategies:** sclerosing agent (silver nitrate), antifibrinolytic agent (tranexamic acid), astringents (alum solution, sucralfate), vasoconstrictive agents [topical oxymetazoline (Afrin®), topical epinephrine]</li></ul>	<ul><li>Consider checking: platelet count, PT/INR, vitamin K deficiency</li><li>Ask: Is transfusion appropriate? Is patient on warfarin? Is the wound infected?</li><li>Atraumatic removal of dressings – irrigate with normal saline to remove dressings</li><li>Use topical vasoconstrictors only when bleeding is minimal, oozing, or seeping</li></ul>
Support Surface	<ul><li>Support surface only if pressure was causative injury leading to ulceration</li></ul>	<ul><li>What is the causative injury?</li></ul>
Pain	**Nonpharmacological Interventions:**<ul><li>**Procedural:** moisture-balanced, non-adherent, long-wear dressings; warm saline irrigation to remove dressings; time-outs; patient participation</li><li>**Complementary therapies:** music, relaxation, aromatherapy, visualization, meditation</li></ul>**Pharmacological Interventions:**<ul><li>**Topical/local:** 2% lidocaine; EMLA® cream; morphine gel</li><li>**Systemic:** scheduled and pre-procedural opioid; tricyclic antidepressant; anticonvulsant</li></ul>	<ul><li>Usually a dull aching pain or heaviness that is relieved as edema decreases - compression or leg elevation decrease edema</li><li>Rule out infection or wound deterioration</li><li>Consider placing: hydrocolloid, foam, calcium alginate, PMD*, soft silicone, or hydrogel</li><li>EMLA® cream is applied to periwound tissue 60 minutes prior to procedure</li><li>Morphine gel is only applied to open/inflamed wounds and must be compounded by a pharmacist</li></ul>

***Cleansers:** Rinse wound bed with normal saline after using antiseptic cleanser to minimize toxic effects **GFD:** Gelling fiber dressing
PMD: polymeric membrane dressing (PolyMem®)   **GV/MB PU Foam:** gentian violet/methylene blue (Hydrofera Blue®Ready™)
NaCl IG: Sodium chloride impregnated gauze (Mesalt®)
Topical Antibiotics: Use of a topical antibiotic is NOT recommended due to the potential for adverse reactions and antimicrobial resistance

Treatment Algorithm for Venous Ulcer

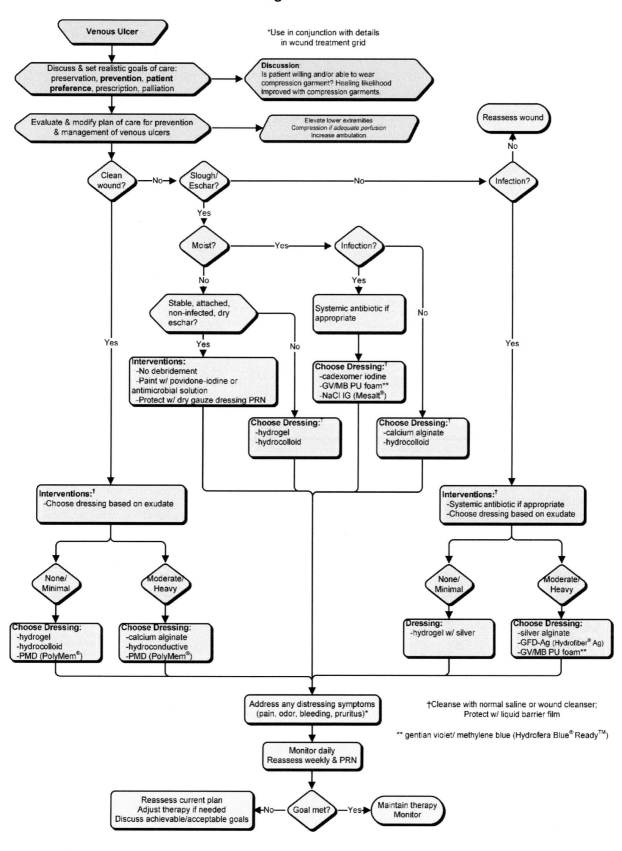

KEY POINTS

- Lower extremity venous disease is caused by venous hypertension as a result of chronic venous insufficiency.
- Compression is the gold standard in the treatment of venous ulcers.
- Dressing selection follows the principles of moist wound healing and the patient's preference for comfort.

CASE STUDY

The nurse is visiting a 70-year-old female patient living in a skilled nursing facility with a primary diagnosis of CHF. While reviewing new orders, the nurse notes treatment orders for a venous ulcer of the right lateral lower extremity. The nurse reviews the facility's wound documentation and notes the following:

Full thickness venous ulcer to the right lateral lower extremity measuring 0.5 x 0.9 cm. Wound bed with 50% slough and 50% granulation tissue. Moderate serous exudate is present. No odor, redness, induration, or edema noted. Surrounding skin is warm, dry, and intact. Numeric pain score 2/10 during wound assessment. ABI is 0.9. Current preventive measures include elevating the lower extremities for 30 minutes four times per day. Comorbidities include hyperlipidemia and hypertension. The patient eats 100% of all meals and ambulates with the assistance of one and a walker. PPS is 50%. The patient and family wish to heal the wound, but the patient prefers not to wear compression. Physician notified of assessment, and new order received: Cleanse venous ulcer right lateral lower extremity with normal saline, pat periwound tissue dry. Apply liquid barrier film to periwound tissue. Apply a gelling fiber dressing (Hydrofiber®) to the wound bed, cover with foam, and secure with Kerlix® gauze. Change every three days and as needed if soiled.

The nurse assesses the wound and listens as the patient and family express frustration because the wound fails to heal despite intensive wound care. The nurse recognizes that compression is the main healing force in venous leg ulcers, not the dressing, and educates the patient and family on the importance of compression in healing venous ulcers. The patient and family again decline the use of compression and agree to the management of symptoms and maintenance as the wound care goal.

In evaluating the outcome, the nurse recognizes that the current treatment orders are in alignment with the wishes and goals of the patient and her family. The nurse will continue to monitor for changes in wound condition or patient's goals that would warrant a change in the plan of care.

References
1. Grey JE, Harding KG, Enoch S. Venous and arterial ulcers. *BMJ*. 2006;332(7537): 347-350. https://www.ncbi.nlm.nih.gov/pmc/articles/PMC1363917/. Accessed May 9, 2017.
2. Takahashi P. Chronic ischemic, venous, and neuropathic ulcers in long-term care. *Ann LTC*. 2006;14(7):26-31.
3. Wound Ostomy and Continence Nurses Society. A quick reference guide for lower-extremity wounds: venous, arterial, and neuropathic. April 4, 2013. http://c.ymcdn.com/sites/www.wocn.org/resource/collection/E3050C1A-FBF0-44ED-B28B-C41E24551CCC/A_Quick_Reference_Guide_for_LE_Wounds_(2013).pdf. Accessed July 14, 2017.
4. Wright J, Richards T, Srai S. The role of iron in the skin and cutaneous wound healing. Front Pharmacol 2014;5:156 https://www.ncbi.nlm.nih.gov/pmc/articles/PMC4091310/ Accessed April 23, 2018

5. Wayne G. Impaired tissue integrity. September 13, 2016 https://nurseslabs.com/impaired-tissue-integrity/ Accessed October 12, 2017.
6. European Wound Management Association (EWMA), Moffat C. Understanding compression therapy. London, UK; Medical Education Partnership LTD, 2003; http://www.woundsinternational.com/pdf/content_51.pdf Accessed April 23, 2018.
7. Kelechi TJ, Johnson JJ. Guideline for the management of wounds in patients with lower-extremity venous disease: an executive summary. *J Wound Ostomy Continence Nurs.* 2012;39(6):598-606
8. Bouza C, Munoz A, Amate J M. Efficacy of modern dressings in the treatment of leg ulcers: a systematic review. *Wound Repair Regen.* 2005;13(3):218-229.
9. Kunimoto BT. Management and prevention of venous leg ulcers: a literature-guided approach. *Ostomy Wound Manage.* 2001;47(6):36-49.
10. American Academy of Dermatology. Statis dermatitis. https://www.aad.org/public/diseases/eczema/stasis-dermatitis Accessed April 23, 2018
11. Sibbald RG, Krasner DL, Lutz J. SCALE: Skin changes at life's end: final consensus statement: October 1, 2009. *Adv Skin Wound Care.* 2010;23(5):225-236.
12. So-Shn Mak S, Lee MY, Cheung JSS, et al. Pressurised irrigation versus swabbing method in cleansing wounds healed by secondary intention: a randomized controlled trial with cost-effectiveness analysis. *Int J Nurs Stud.* 2015;52:88-101.
13. Hofman D. The autolytic debridement of venous leg ulcers. *Wound Essentials.* 2007;2:68-73. http://www.woundsinternational.com/media/issues/221/files/content_186.pdf Accessed May 11, 2017.
14. Ramundo J. Wound debridement. In Bryant RA, Nix DP, eds. Acute & Chronic Wounds: Current Management Concepts. 4th ed. St. Louis, MO:Elsevier/Mosby;2012:279-288.
15. Rolstad BS, Bryant RA, Nix DP. Topical management. In Bryant RA, Nix DP, eds. *Acute & Chronic Wounds: Current Management Concepts.* 4th ed. St Louis, MO:Elsevier/Mosby;2012:289-306.
16. Popescu A, Sal Salcido R. Wound pain: a challenge for the patient and the wound care specialist. *Adv Skin Wound Care.* 2004;17(1):14-20.
17. Tran QNH, Fancher T. Achieving analgesia for painful ulcers using topically applied morphine gel. *J Support Oncol.* 2007;5(6):289-293.

DIABETIC FOOT ULCERS

GOALS

Within the confines of the patient's prognosis and in alignment with the wishes of the patient and family:

- Maintain skin integrity with individualized prevention strategies
- Preserve existing areas of ulceration to prevent infection and gangrene
- Relieve distressing symptoms and promote quality of life

DEFINITIONS

A **diabetic foot ulcer** is an ulceration that presents on the foot of a diabetic patient. Diabetic foot ulcers fall into three categories: neuropathic, ischemic, and neuroischemic. The **neuropathic diabetic foot ulcer** is secondary to **lower extremity neuropathic disease (LEND)**. An individual with lower extremity neuropathic disease will demonstrate sensory, motor, and autonomic neuropathy. Sensory neuropathy leads to the loss of sensation in the foot putting the patient at risk of injury from trauma. Motor neuropathy leads to deformities of the foot placing the patient at risk of abnormal pressure to the bony prominences of the foot, callus formation, and subsequent ulceration. Autonomic neuropathy results in a reduction of oil and moisture to the

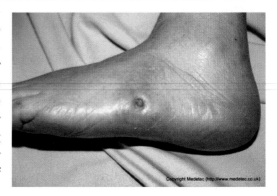

Figure 3. Diabetic Foot Ulcer

foot, which will manifest as dry skin that may peel or fissure, placing the patient at risk of developing an infection. Diabetic foot ulcers are also associated with lower extremity arterial disease, either purely ischemic (**ischemic diabetic foot ulcers**) or a combination of neuropathy and ischemia (**neuroischemic diabetic foot ulcers**).[1]

ASSESSMENT

Diagnose neuropathic diabetic foot ulcers based on distinguishing characteristics (*see Table 4*).[1-3] Identify neuropathy using the monofilament test and tuning fork. An Ankle Brachial Index rules out ischemic and neuroischemic ulcers in the diabetic patient population. An Ankle Brachial Index of 0.90 or less indicates that arterial disease is present; however, the Ankle Brachial Index can be greater than 1.30 in the diabetic patient, which means that the arteries of the ankle are calcified. If this occurs, obtain a Toe Brachial Index (TBI). The TBI is equal to the toe systolic pressure divided by the brachial systolic pressure. A TBI less than 0.64 indicates that arterial disease is present.[2]

Use the Wagner classification system to grade the severity of the diabetic foot ulcer. This classification system assigns a grade ranging from 0 (no ulcers present) to 5 (gangrene of the entire foot) by evaluating ulcer depth, presence of gangrene, and loss of perfusion.[1]

Table 4. Presentation of Diabetic Foot Ulcers[1-3]			
Characteristic	Neuropathic	Ischemic	Neuroischemic
Location	• Plantar surface of foot • Areas of the foot that bear weight – heel, ball of the foot, great toe	• Margins of the feet and toes • Tips of toes	• Margins of the feet and toes • Tips of toes • Under thickened toe nails
Etiology	• Neuropathy (assess using the monofilament test and tuning fork) with unrecognized pressure to bony prominences or trauma as sources of injury	• Ischemia from lower extremity arterial disease with trauma as a source of injury (e.g., poorly fitted shoes)	• Combination of neuropathic changes of the foot and ischemia from lower extremity arterial disease
Wound Bed	• May be hidden under thick callus or have callus around perimeter • Pink; granulation tissue possible • Round and "punched out"	• May present as a blister • Necrosis likely • Pale in color • Granulation reduced/absent	• May present as a red area • If callus is present, may be minimal • Necrosis possible • Granulation reduced/absent
Appearance of Foot	• Dry, flakey skin, fissures • Deformities • Warm	• Cool • Pulses absent • Thin, shiny, hairless skin	• Cool • Pulses absent • Thin, shiny, hairless skin
Pain	• Usually painless due to numbness and loss of sensation	• Painful	• May be present or absent

PLAN OF CARE

Develop an individualized plan of care to prevent the development of or treat existing diabetic foot ulcers to guide the actions of all members of the interdisciplinary team. The care plan serves to translate the data gained from completion of the comprehensive assessment into a specific plan of action to prevent or manage diabetic foot ulcers. Table 5 includes potential care plans for diabetic foot ulcers.[3,4]

Table 5. Plan of Care for Diabetic Foot Ulcers		
Nursing Diagnosis	Related Factors	Interventions
Risk for Impaired Skin Integrity • Patient has the potential for an alteration in skin integrity **Impaired Skin Integrity** • Partial thickness tissue loss **Impaired Tissue Integrity** • Full thickness tissue loss	• Advanced age • Alcohol abuse • Chemotherapy • Diabetes • Pressure • Cardiovascular disease • Lower extremity arterial disease • Kidney disease • Smoking • Knowledge deficit • Trauma	• Assess skin, note areas of discoloration, texture, or temperature and any existing skin alterations • Relieve pain if present • Revascularization surgery if ischemia is present • Maintain adequate nutrition and hydration • Offload pressure and assist with ambulation • Protect from lower extremities from trauma – monitor lower extremities and feet daily • Assess skin alteration and determine etiology, reassess regularly, monitor daily • Diabetic foot care • Localized wound care, prevent/treat infection

INTERVENTIONS

Prevention
Diabetic foot ulcers are undesirable because they fail to heal and often become infected. Gangrene and the subsequent necessity for amputation are also possible. Therefore, prevention of the diabetic foot ulcer should continue to be a focus for the palliative care patient. Instruct the patient to:[3]

- Check feet daily – both looking and feeling
- Wash feet with warm water and dry thoroughly (even between the toes)
- Apply moisturizer to the feet but never between the toes
- Ensure socks and shoes fit well – not too loose or too tight
- When ambulating, shoes should always be worn – never barefoot
- Cut toenails straight across
- Rotate shoes throughout the day to vary the pressure on the feet
- Refrain from soaking the feet or self-trimming a callus (may use a pumice stone)
- Protect the feet from trauma while in bed (e.g., float heels), during transfers from bed (e.g., sheepskin or foam boots), and while ambulating (e.g., good-fitting shoes, offload pressure with assistive devices)

Localized Wound Care
Treatment of the diabetic foot ulcer varies based on the underlying cause. If ischemia is present, revascularization of the leg may be necessary to achieve wound healing. Tight glycemic control, smoking cessation, and maximizing nutrition are critical. The source of trauma needs to be reversed, whether it is from ill-fitting footwear, deformities of the foot, or the presence of a foreign body. The pressure of the foot must be offloaded, usually through the use of a total contact cast or assistive devices. The callus will need debridement, with sharp debridement being the method of choice. If gangrene is present, amputation is a possible outcome. Collectively, these treatment options impose significant burden on the patient and may not be practical at the end of life. Therefore, for the palliative management of the diabetic foot ulcer, the primary goal will be the prevention of infection and symptom management. Principles of moist wound healing and wound bed preparation will govern the dressing selection for the neuropathic diabetic foot ulcer.[3,5] Conversely, principles of dry wound healing will govern dressing selection if ischemia is severe and wound healing is unlikely.[6,7] Use the following algorithms and treatment grids to assist in selecting an appropriate dressing.

WOUND TREATMENT GRID: Diabetic Foot Ulcers[1-3,5-10]		
Wound Need	**Intervention**	**Comments**
Cleanse	• **Clean wound bed:** pour normal saline or wound cleanser • **Infection/necrosis:** irrigate with wound cleanser or antiseptic*	• Irrigate with 4-15 psi: piston syringe (4.2 psi), squeeze bottle+irrigation cap(4.5 psi), 35 mL syringe+18 gauge needle (8 psi)
Debridement	• **Dry:** hydrogel, hydrocolloid • **Moist:** calcium alginate, hydrocolloid, hydroconductive • **Infected:** silver alginate, cadexomer iodine, hydroconductive	• Neuropathic: Sharp debridement of callus. • Ischemia: Debridement is NOT recommended unless perfusion status is known. See *Arterial Ulcer Algorithm*, page 65
Exudate	• **None/Minimal Exudate:** hydrogel, hydrocolloid, PMD* • **Moderate Exudate:** foam, calcium alginate, PMD* • **Heavy Exudate:** GFD* (Hydrofiber®), hydroconductive, PMD* • **Stable eschar:** paint perimeter with povidone-iodine	• Monitor daily – rapid deterioration of the wound is possible • Cautious use of occlusive dressings • PMDs* can be used on all exudate levels – moisten with saline if wound bed is dry
Infection	• **None/Minimal Exudate:** honey, hydrogel with silver • **Moderate Exudate:** silver alginate, honey alginate, silver foam • **Heavy Exudate:** GFD* (Hydrofiber®) with silver, cadexomer iodine, hydroconductive	• Decreased inflammatory response so only subtle signs of an infection may be present • Can lead to gangrene; rule out osteomyelitis • Systemic antibiotics are necessary – wound culture guides selection*
Malodor	• **Cleansers*:** hypochlorous acid (Vashe®), sodium hypochlorite (Dakin's® 0.125%) • **Dressings:** cadexomer iodine, honey, charcoal, silver, essential oils (wintergreen or lavender) on dressing • **Environmental strategies:** kitty litter, vanilla extract, coffee grounds, or dryer sheets placed in room	• Rule our infection • Wound cleansing aids odor control. • Change dressing more often to manage odor (e.g., hydrocolloid every 24-48 hours). • Hydrocolloid dressings tend to create odor (doesn't mean infection is present)
Dead Space	• **None/Minimal Exudate:** hydrogel, PMD* • **Moderate Exudate:** foam, calcium alginate, PMD* • **Heavy Exudate:** GFD* (Hydrofiber®), hydroconductive, PMD*	• Loosely fill any dead space. • Products are available in different forms, such as roping, to pack tunnels
Pruritus	• Not usually associated with the wound, assess surrounding skin.	• Evaluate for contact dermatitis, hypersensitivity, or yeast dermatitis
Bleeding	• **Dressing strategies:** calcium alginate (silver alginate is not hemostatic), non-adherent dressing, or coagulants (gelatin sponge, thrombin) • **Topical/local strategies:** sclerosing agent (silver nitrate), antifibrinolytic agent (tranexamic acid), astringents (alum solution, sucralfate), vasoconstrictive agents [topical oxymetazoline (Afrin®), topical epinephrine]	• Atraumatic removal of dressings – irrigate with normal saline to remove dressings • Ask: Is transfusion appropriate? Is patient on warfarin? Is the wound infected? • Consider checking: platelet count, PT/INR, vitamin K deficiency • Use topical vasoconstrictors only when bleeding is minimal, oozing, or seeping
Support Surface	• Consider the need for a support surface if pressure was causative injury leading to ulceration	• What was the causative injury?
Pain	**Nonpharmacological Interventions:** • **Procedural:** moisture-balanced, non-adherent dressings; warm saline irrigation to remove dressings; time-outs; patient participation • **Complementary therapies:** music, relaxation, aromatherapy, visualization, meditation **Pharmacological Interventions:** • **Systemic:** scheduled and pre-procedural opioid; tricyclic antidepressant; anticonvulsant	• Rule out infection and wound deterioration • Neuropathic diabetic foot ulcers can be painless due to loss of sensation • Consider placing: hydrocolloid, foam, calcium alginate, PMD*, soft silicone, or hydrogel
***Cleansers:** Rinse wound bed with normal saline after using antiseptic cleanser to minimize toxic effects ‖**GFD:** Gelling fiber dressing **PMD:** polymeric membrane dressing (PolyMem®) **Topical Antibiotics:** Use of a topical antibiotic is NOT recommended due to the potential for adverse reactions and antimicrobial resistance		

Treatment Algorithm for Diabetic Foot Ulcer

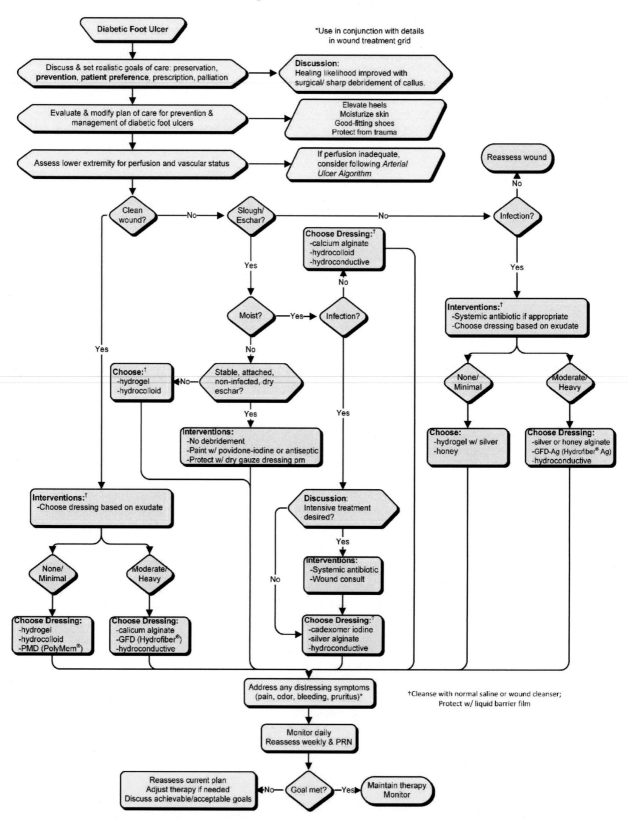

KEY POINTS

- Diabetic foot ulcers are defined as any skin alteration in the foot of the diabetic patient. They fall into three categories: neuropathic, ischemic, and neuroischemic.
- Because diabetic foot ulcers are associated with a decrease in quality of life, prevention strategies should continue in the palliative care population.
- Principles of moist wound healing and wound bed preparation will govern the dressing selection for the neuropathic diabetic foot ulcer.

CASE STUDY

The nurse is admitting a 64-year-old male patient to hospice with a primary diagnosis of malignant melanoma. While performing a head to toe assessment, the nurse notes a diabetic ulcer to the plantar surface of the right great toe. The nurse performs a comprehensive wound assessment and documents the following:

Full thickness diabetic neuropathic ulcer to the plantar surface of the right great toe measuring 1.3 x 1.9 x 0.7 cm. Wound bed with 100% granulation tissue. Callus surrounds the perimeter of the wound. Moderate serous exudate. No odor, redness, induration, or edema noted. Surrounding tissue is warm, dry, and intact. Numeric pain score 2/10 during wound assessment. ABI is 0.8, and capillary refill is within normal limits. The patient denies the use of any prevention strategies at this time. The patient reports having custom orthotic shoes but stopped wearing them after being diagnosed with cancer. Comorbidities include hyperlipidemia and hypertension. The patient is taking comfort medications only. The patient eats approximately 75% of all meals and weight is stable at 182 pounds. The patient ambulates independently. PPS is 50%. The patient does not wish to pursue intensive treatment for this wound, including surgical/sharp debridement of callus. The family currently cares for the wound by washing daily with soap and water and applying a gauze dressing.

The nurse educates the patient and family on preventive strategies for diabetic foot ulcers to prevent further injury to the patient's feet. The nurse suggests discontinuing the gauze dressing because this places the patient at increased risk of developing an infection. Instead, the nurse recommends an absorptive dressing. The nurse notifies the physician of her assessment and recommendations. The physician agrees with the nurse's assessment and provides the following wound care orders:

- Cleanse diabetic foot ulcer plantar surface of the right great toe with normal saline. Pat periwound tissue dry. Loosely fill dead space with calcium alginate and cover with a foam dressing. Secure with tape. Change every three days and as needed if soiled.

The nurse reviews the wound care orders with the family, and the family is agreeable to the plan of care. The nurse provides education regarding the application of the dressing. The patient and family return-demonstrate the procedure.

References

1. Wounds International. *Best Practice Guidelines: Wound Management in Diabetic Foot Ulcers.* London, UK:Wounds Int'l; 2013. http://www.woundsinternational.com/media/best-practices/_/673/files/dfubestpracticeforweb.pdf Accessed April 23, 2018

2. Wound Ostomy and Continence Nurses Society. A quick reference guide for lower-extremity wounds: venous, arterial, and neuropathic. April 4, 2013. http://c.ymcdn.com/sites/www.wocn.org/resource/collection/E3050C1A-FBF0-44ED-B28B-C41E24551CCC/A_Quick_Reference_Guide_for_LE_Wounds_(2013).pdf Accessed July 14, 2017.

3. Heitzman, J. Foot care for patients with diabetes. *Top Geriatr Rehabil.* 2010;26(3):250-263.

4. Wayne G. Impaired tissue integrity. September 13, 2016 https://nurseslabs.com/impaired-tissue-integrity/ Accessed October 12, 2017.

5. Edmonds, ME, Foster AVM. ABC of wound healing: diabetic foot ulcers. *BMJ.* 2006;332:407-410.

6. Takahashi P. Chronic ischemic, venous, and neuropathic ulcers in long-term care. *Ann LTC.* 2006;14(7):26-31.

7. Williams RL. Cadexomer iodine: an effective palliative dressing in chronic critical limb ischemia. *Wounds.* 2009;21(1):15-28.

8. So-Shn Mak S, Lee MY, Cheung JSS, et al. Pressurized irrigation versus swabbing method in cleansing wounds healed by secondary intention: a randomized controlled trial with cost-effectiveness analysis. *Int J Nurs Stud.* 2015;52:88-101.

9. Sibbald RG, Krasner DL, Lutz J. SCALE: Skin changes at life's end: final consensus statement: October 1, 2009. *Adv Skin Wound Care.* 2010;23(5):225-236.

10. Popescu A, Sal Salcido R. Wound pain: a challenge for the patient and the wound care specialist. *Adv Skin Wound Care.* 2004;17(1):14-20.

SKIN TEARS

GOALS

Within the confines of the patient's prognosis and in alignment with the wishes of the patient and family:

- Prevent injury with individualized prevention strategies
- Provide localized wound care with non-adherent dressings that maintain a moist wound bed.
- Relieve distressing symptoms and promote quality of life

DEFINITIONS

A **skin tear** is the separation of skin layers as a result of trauma or from exposure to friction or shear. Skin tears occur primarily on the extremities. They may be partial or full thickness injuries. A **partial thickness skin tear** is the separation of the epidermis from the dermis, while a **full thickness skin tear** is the separation of the epidermis and dermis from the underlying subcutaneous tissue.[1]

ASSESSMENT

A comprehensive skin assessment is the first step in preventing and treating skin tears. Use the International Skin Tear Advisory Panel's skin tear risk assessment when conducting a skin assessment. This risk assessment assists in implementing preventive strategies for those patients who are at risk or high risk of developing a skin tear. Risk factors for the development of skin tears include the presence of advanced disease, polypharmacy, impaired senses, poor cognition, altered nutritional status, impaired mobility, dependence on activities of daily living, advanced age, delicate skin, and a history of falls or skin tears. The presence of one risk factor places the patient at risk. Implement preventive strategies.[1]

Assess skin tears, at a minimum, weekly, and more frequently with a change in the patient's condition except when the patient is imminently dying. Classify skin tears using the classification system developed by the International Skin Tear Advisory Panel. These classifications are as follows:[1]

- Type 1: Linear skin tear or a skin tear with a flap that can be replaced over the entire wound bed
- Type 2: Skin tear in which the part of the flap is lost and cannot cover the entire wound bed
- Type 3: Skin tear in which the flap is completely lost, and the entire wound bed is exposed

PLAN OF CARE

Develop an individualized plan of care for the prevention and treatment of skin tears to guide the actions of all members of the interdisciplinary team. The care plan will serve to translate the data gained from completion of the comprehensive assessment and risk assessment into a specific plan of action to prevent and manage these injuries. Table 1 includes potential care plans for skin tears.[1,8]

Table 1. Plan of Care for Skin Tears		
Nursing Diagnosis	**Related Factors**	**Interventions**
Risk for Impaired Skin Integrity • Patient has the potential for an alteration in skin integrity **Impaired Skin Integrity** • Partial thickness tissue loss **Impaired Tissue Integrity** • Full thickness tissue loss	• Presence of advanced disease • Polypharmacy • Impaired senses • Poor cognition • Altered nutritional status • Impaired mobility • Dependence on activities of daily living • Advanced age • Frail skin • History of falls or skin tears	• Assess skin, note areas of discoloration, texture, or temperature and any existing skin alterations • Develop a safe patient environment (fall prevention, clutter-free area, adequate room lighting, pad furniture, correct use of assistive devices) • Use protective clothing, do NOT wear sharp jewelry • Review medications for polypharmacy/fall risk • Safe patient handling and assistance • Trim nails • Maintain skin clean and dry • Avoid the use of adhesives • Maximize nutrition and hydration, consult dietician • Assess skin alteration, determine etiology, monitor daily • Localized wound care

INTERVENTIONS

Prevention

Skin tears are painful and decrease the quality of life for any patient. Therefore, prevention of skin tears is the primary intervention. Prevent skin tears by:[1]

- Creating a safe patient environment. Ensure the area has adequate lighting and is clutter-free. Pad furniture as needed. Initiate fall prevention strategies.
- Encouraging the patient to keep nails trimmed short, refrain from wearing jewelry with sharp edges, and wear protective clothing (e.g., long-sleeved shirts).
- Ensuring the patient uses assistive devices correctly.
- Maximizing nutrition and hydration status. Consult a dietician as needed.
- Promoting safe patient handling techniques: provide assistance with mobility and transfers, maintain skin clean and dry, and refrain from using adhesives.
- Conducting a medication review to identify medications that increase the risk of falls or instances of polypharmacy. Adjust the medication regimen as needed.

Localized Wound Care

When treating a skin tear, use non-adherent dressings that promote a moist wound bed while minimizing pain, preventing infection, and offering a long wear time.[9] Secure dressings with tubular netting or gauze rolls to minimize placing tape on the patient's fragile skin. Note that the International Skin Tear Advisory Panel recommends skin glue to approximate wound edges for Type 1 skin tears; however, the use of skin glue may be limited due to potential product availability issues in the home setting and the need for a medical directive. If a skin tear fails to heal, particularly a skin tear of a lower extremity, consider the underlying disease process that may act as a barrier to healing (e.g., lower extremity arterial disease). Use the following algorithm and treatment grid to assist in selecting an appropriate dressing.

WOUND TREATMENT GRID: Skin Tears[1-7,9,10]		
Wound Need	**Intervention**	**Comments**
Cleanse	• **Clean wound bed:** pour normal saline or wound cleanser • **Infection/necrosis/foreign bodies:** irrigate with wound cleanser or antiseptic*	• Irrigate with 4-15 psi: piston syringe (4.2 psi), squeeze bottle +irrigation cap (4.5 psi), or 35 mL syringe+18 gauge needle (8 psi)
Debridement	• **Dry:** hydrogel • **Moist:** foam, calcium alginate • **Infected:** silver hydrogel, silver foam, silver alginate	• Rare, consider underlying etiology if slough or eschar is present • Irrigate the wound to remove foreign bodies
Exudate	• **None/Minimal Exudate:** petrolatum, petrolatum/3% Bismuth tribromophenate (Xeroform™) gauze, hydrogel • **Moderate/Heavy Exudate:** non-adherent foam (PMD*), calcium alginate, or GFD* (Hydrofiber®) • Use non-adherent gauze pads as secondary dressings	• Protect periwound: apply skin barrier film • Replace skin flap before placing dressing • Use non-stick gauze, tubular netting, or gauze roll to secure dressings; limit frequency of dressing changes unless necessary
Infection	• **None/Minimal Exudate:** silver hydrogel • **Moderate Exudate/Heavy Exudate:** silver foam (PMD* with silver), silver alginate, GFD* (Hydrofiber®) with silver	May treat infection empirically: • MRSA: cadexomer iodine, mupirocin*, silver • Pseudomonas: cadexomer iodine, acetic acid • VRE: GV/MB PU foam*, silver • MSSA: cadexomer iodine, chlorhexidine, GV/MB PU foam*, mupirocin*, silver
Malodor	• **Cleansers*:** hypochlorous acid (Vashe®), sodium hypochlorite (Dakin's® 0.125%), acetic acid (0.25-0.5%) • **Dressings:** cadexomer iodine, honey, charcoal, silver, metronidazole (Flagyl®) to wound bed, essential oils (wintergreen or lavender) on dressing • **Environmental strategies:** kitty litter, vanilla extract, coffee grounds, dryer sheets placed in room	• Rule out infection • Wound cleansing aids odor control. • Change dressing more often to manage odor
Dead Space	• Loosely fill dead space with the products listed above	• Products are available in different forms, such as roping
Pruritus	• Not usually associated with wound, assess surrounding skin and consider wound care product being used	• Evaluate for contact dermatitis, hypersensitivity, or yeast dermatitis
Bleeding	• **Dressing strategies:** calcium alginate (silver alginate is not hemostatic), non-adherent dressing, or coagulants (gelatin sponge, thrombin) • **Topical/local strategies:** sclerosing agent (silver nitrate), antifibrinolytic agent (tranexamic acid), astringents (alum solution, sucralfate), vasoconstrictive agents [topical oxymetazoline (Afrin®), topical epinephrine]	• Atraumatic removal of dressings – irrigate with normal saline to remove dressings. • Ask: Is the wound infected? Is patient on warfarin? Is transfusion appropriate? • Consider checking: platelet count, PT/INR, vitamin K deficiency • Use topical vasoconstrictors only when bleeding is minimal, oozing, or seeping
Support Surface	• Consider the need for a support surface only if a pressure injury is present.	• What was the causative injury?
Pain	**Nonpharmacological Interventions:** • **Procedural:** moisture-balanced, non-adherent, long-wear dressings; warm saline irrigation to remove dressings; time-outs; patient participation • **Complementary therapies:** music, relaxation, aromatherapy, visualization, meditation **Pharmacological Interventions:** • **Topical/local:** 2% lidocaine; EMLA® cream • **Systemic:** scheduled and pre-procedural opioid; tricyclic antidepressant; anticonvulsant	• Rule out infection or wound deterioration • Consider placing: foam, calcium alginate, PMD*, soft silicone, or hydrogel • EMLA® cream is applied to periwound tissue 60 minutes before the procedure

***Cleansers:** Rinse wound bed with normal saline after using antiseptic cleanser to minimize toxic effects ‖**GFD:** Gelling fiber dressing
PMD: polymeric membrane dressing (PolyMem®) **GV/MB PU Foam:** gentian violet/methylene blue (Hydrofera Blue®Ready™)
Topical Antibiotics: Use of a topical antibiotic is NOT recommended due to the potential for adverse reactions and antimicrobial resistance

Treatment Algorithm for Acute Skin Tear

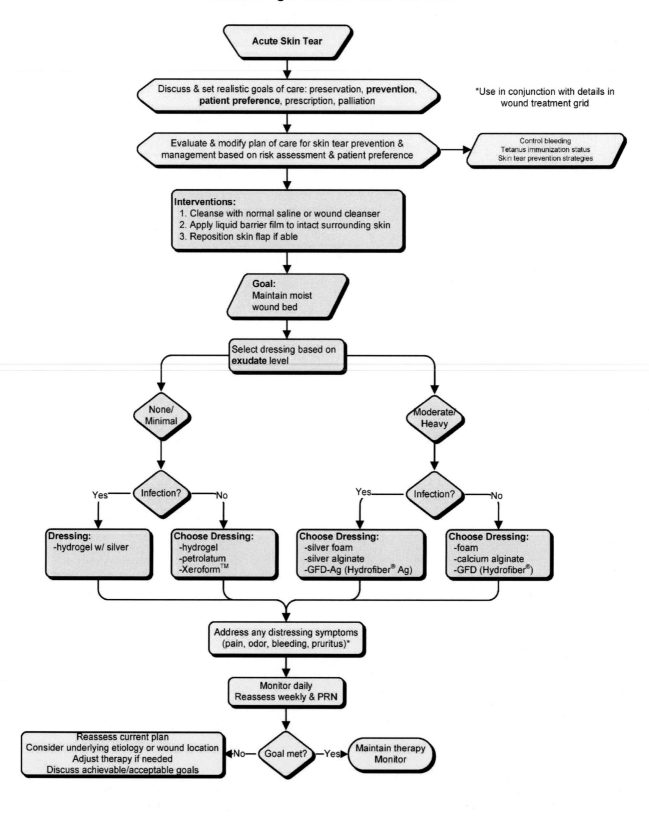

KEY POINTS

- Because skin tears are preventable and associated with a decrease in quality of life, prevention strategies should continue in the palliative care population.
- Principles of moist wound healing and wound bed preparation will govern the dressing selection for the skin tear with an emphasis on selecting a non-adherent dressing.

CASE STUDY

The emergency on-call nurse is evaluating a 77-year-old male patient living with his family with a primary diagnosis of Parkinson's disease. The patient fell while trying to ambulate to the restroom. The patient's only injury is a skin tear on the right forearm measuring 3.1 x 2.5.x 0.1 cm. The entire skin flap is intact. No active bleeding noted at this time. The wound bed has light serous drainage. After notifying the physician and receiving orders, the nurse irrigates the wound with normal saline to remove foreign bodies, repositions the skin flap to cover the wound bed, and applies liquid skin barrier film to the periwound tissue. The nurse then applies petrolatum gauze to the wound bed and secures it with a non-stick dressing and rolled gauze. The nurse educates the family on the application of the dressing and instructs them to change the dressing every three days and PRN if soiled. Because the skin tear is related to a fall, the nurse also investigates the cause of the fall. The patient states that his walker became entangled in a floor rug. The family removes floor rugs, and the nurse modifies the plan of care to reflect this change.

References

1. LeBlanc K, Baranoski S, Alam T, et al. Evidence based prediction, prevention, assessment, and management of skin tears. International Skin Tear Advisory Panel (ISTAP) http://www.skintears.org/education/tools/skin-tear-tool-kit/ Accessed September 27, 2017.
2. Ramundo J. Wound debridement. In Bryant RA, Nix DP, eds. *Acute & Chronic Wounds: Current Management Concepts.* 4th ed. St Louis, MO:Elsevier/Mosby;2012:279-288.
3. Sibbald RG, Krasner DL, Lutz J. SCALE: Skin changes at life's end: final consensus statement. *Adv Skin Wound Care.* 2010;23(5):225-236.
4. Rolstad BS, Bryant RA, Nix DP. Topical management. In Bryant RA, Nix DP, eds. *Acute & Chronic Wounds: Current Management Concepts.* 4th ed. St Louis, MO:Elsevier/Mosby;2012: 289-306.
5. Hopf HW, Shapshak D, Junkins S. Managing wound pain. In Bryant RA, Nix DP, eds. *Acute & Chronic Wounds: Current Management Concepts.* 4th ed. St Louis, MO:Elsevier/Mosby;2012: 380-387.
6. Tran QNH, Fancher T. Achieving analgesia for painful ulcers using topically applied morphine gel. *J Support Oncol* 2007;5(6):289-293.
7. Popescu A, Sal Salcido R. Wound pain: a challenge for the patient and the wound care specialist. *Adv Skin Wound Care.* 2004;17(1):14-20.
8. Wayne G. Impaired tissue integrity. September 13, 2016 https://nurseslabs.com/impaired-tissue-integrity/ Accessed October 12, 2017.
9. Moser L. Skin tears: keeping it together. *Ostomy Wound Manage.* 2011;57(3):10. http://www.o-wm.com/files/owm/pdfs/March_Pearls.pdf. Accessed October 16, 2017.
10. So-Shn Mak S, Lee MY, Cheung JSS, et al. Pressurised irrigation versus swabbing method in cleansing wounds healed by secondary intention: a randomized controlled trial with cost-effectiveness analysis. *Int J Nurs Stud.* 2015;52:88-101.

FUNGATING (MALIGNANT) WOUNDS

GOALS

Within the confines of the patient's prognosis and in alignment with the wishes of the patient and family:

- Assist the patient and family in developing realistic goals of care
- Relieve distressing symptoms
- Promote independence and quality of life

DEFINITIONS

A **fungating** or **malignant wound** is the manifestation of malignant cells that have infiltrated the skin and associated structures, such as blood and lymphatic vessels. Although rare, malignant wounds are most likely to occur with primary tumors of the breast, lung, skin, or gastrointestinal tract. Fungating wounds initially present as discolored nodules under the surface of the skin. As the lesion grows, it penetrates the skin. Oxygen deprivation leads to cell death and tissue necrosis. This lack of oxygen and tissue necrosis also provides an ideal environment for the proliferation of anaerobic bacteria, which gives malignant wounds their characteristic odor and exudate. Over time, the fungating wound will protrude above the level of the skin or form an ulceration that appears as a crater within the skin. Lymphedema is present if the tumor infiltrates the lymphatic system.[1]

ASSESSMENT

Fungating wounds are a source of psychosocial distress for the patient. Not only are they a visible reminder of an often fatal disease process, but they can also limit independence and cause embarrassment or social isolation due to their malodor and exudate. Evaluate the impact of the wound on the independence, social status, living environment, social support, and self-care of the patient and their family/caregiver. Also assess for symptoms that frequently accompany these wounds, including pain, bleeding, exudate, odor, and infection by recognizing local wound conditions that contribute to symptom development. Healing is not the goal for these wounds; therefore, when providing localized wound interventions, assess the outcome of these interventions based on the improvement of the patient's quality of life and independence. All decisions regarding wound care should incorporate the patient's preference.[1,2]

PLAN OF CARE

Develop an individualized plan of care for the management of fungating wounds that focuses on the implementation of palliative measures. A well-developed plan of care will include the input of the entire interdisciplinary team. Table 1 includes potential care plans for malignant wounds.[1,3]

Table 1. Plan of Care for Malignant Wounds		
Nursing Diagnosis	**Related Factors**	**Interventions**
Risk for Impaired Skin Integrity • Patient has the potential for an alteration in skin integrity	• Presence of advanced disease (malignancy)	• Assess skin, note areas of discoloration, texture, or temperature and any existing skin alterations • Assess skin alteration and determine etiology • Localized wound care • Monitor daily • Address distressing symptoms (e.g., bleeding, odor, pain, pruritus, exudate)
Impaired Skin Integrity • Partial thickness tissue loss		
Impaired Tissue Integrity • Full thickness tissue loss		

INTERVENTIONS

Provide patient-specific, localized wound care tailored to meet the unique conditions of the wound. Because the characteristics of the wound are ever evolving, adjust the interventions over time to continue to provide comfort and quality of life. Healing is not realistic, and interventions should address the prevention or management of symptoms.

Bleeding
Bleeding is possible with a malignant wound and can range in severity from slow capillary bleeding to hemorrhaging. Prevention of bleeding is an important wound care goal. Prevention strategies include:[1]

- Cleansing with gentle irrigation rather than swabbing.
- Applying non-adherent dressings to prevent trauma to the wound bed during dressing removal. Use contact layers, petrolatum gauze, or petrolatum/3% Bismuth Tribromophenate (Xeroform™) gauze as the primary dressing.
- Removing dressings by gentle irrigation with normal saline.
- Review medication profile for any drug or supplement that might have anti-coagulant or anti-platelet effects or otherwise increase the risk of bleeding.

If bleeding ensues, select one of the following strategies:[1,4]

- Apply pressure, as tolerated by the patient, for 10 to 15 minutes with plain gauze, gauze soaked with topical vasoconstrictive agents [topical oxymetazoline (Afrin®), topical epinephrine], or gauze soaked with tranexamic acid (500 milligrams in 5 milliliters).
- Apply ice packs.
- Apply hemostatic agents, such as gelatin sponges, topical thrombin, calcium alginate, collagen dressings, or Quikclot®. Apply these under pressure if necessary.
- Cauterize small areas of bleeding with silver nitrate.

Hemorrhaging is possible and poses a threat to life. Discuss the potential for this with the patient, and guide interventions based on the wishes of the patient. If the patient wishes to remain in the home, initiate comfort measures, such as using dark towels and medicating for pain and anxiety as needed.

Pain
Manage pain in the fungating tumor using both nonpharmacological and pharmacological interventions. Potential nonpharmacological interventions include the use of moisture-balanced, non-adherent, long-wear dressings, gentle irrigation with warm saline to cleanse the wound and remove dressings, procedural

time-outs, and patient participation where possible. Attempt complimentary therapies, such as music, relaxation, aromatherapy, visualization, and meditation. Pharmacological interventions include both topical and systemic medications. Topical pharmacological interventions include the use of 2% lidocaine at least three minutes before wound care, or EMLA® cream 30 to 60 minutes before wound care, to reduce wound pain.[5,6] Use morphine in hydrogel for open, inflamed wounds.[7] Systemic pharmacological interventions include the use of scheduled and pre-procedural opioid or tricyclic antidepressant and anticonvulsants to address nociceptive and neuropathic wound pain.[5]

Odor and Infection

Odor is a distressing symptom of fungating wounds. The odor is thought to arise from the proliferation of anaerobic bacteria in the necrotic tissue, from volatile fatty acids, pooling exudate, infection, or the presence of a fistula (see Special Topics, page 103). Odor related to the proliferation of anaerobic bacteria within the necrotic tissue may be reduced with the application of metronidazole directly on to the wound bed after cleansing. If the wound is dry, use metronidazole gel. If the wound is moist, use metronidazole powder. Topical metronidazole may take up to three days to control odor or may fail to resolve odor in wounds that are difficult to access, such as vaginal or perineal tumors; consider the use of systemic metronidazole. Use topical antimicrobial dressings, such as cadexomer iodine or silver products, to treat odor related to multi-organism infection. For deeper or systemic infections, use systemic antibiotics and topical antimicrobials.[1]

Removal of necrotic tissue using autolytic or enzymatic debridement can also help to reduce odor to a tolerable level. Use dressings, such as hydrocolloids (light exudate), calcium alginate (moderate exudate), gelling fiber dressings, or sodium chloride impregnated gauze (heavy exudate) for autolytic debridement. Apply collagenase (Santyl®) directly to the wound bed daily for enzymatic debridement.[1]

Use charcoal dressings to neutralize offensive odors. Indications and instructions for the use of charcoal dressings vary by type and manufacturer. Therefore, review the manufacturer's instructions before placing a charcoal dressing. Seal the perimeter of the charcoal dressing to maximize effectiveness with the understanding that this may or may not be possible depending upon the condition of the periwound skin. Other strategies for controlling wound odor include the use of antiseptics, such as Dakin's® solution, hypochlorous acid solution (Vashe®), or acetic acid to cleanse the wound; increasing the frequency of the dressing changes; or placing kitty litter, essential oils, coffee grounds, or dryer sheets in the room.[1]

Exudate

Excessive exudate can cause patient distress at the end of life by causing leakage and painful, frequent dressing changes. Manage exudate by matching the topical dressing to the level of exudate. For low levels of exudate, keep the wound bed moist with impregnated gauze or hydrogel. For moderate exudate, use foam or calcium alginate. For heavily exudating wounds, use super absorbent dressings, such as gelling fiber dressings or specialty absorptives. Use pouching systems to collect the exudate if dressings fail to control the exudate.[1]

Cosmetic Appeal

The cosmetic appearance of a wound can be a source of embarrassment for the palliative patient.[8] Therefore, develop methods of concealing the wound so that it is cosmetically acceptable to the patient. Possible ways of making a wound dressing cosmetically acceptable include:

- Choosing dressings that are the same color as the skin tone of the patient.[8]
- Applying dressings to make the body appear symmetrical.[8]
- Avoiding overly bulky dressings.[1,8]
- Using clothing to secure dressings when possible.

WOUND TREATMENT GRID: Malignant Wounds[1,2,4-10]

Wound Need	Intervention	Comments
Cleanse	• Gently irrigate, avoid swabbing the wound; normal saline preferred to minimize pain; antiseptics if odor is problematic*	• Gentle irrigation minimizes risk of acute bleeding
Debridement	• **Dry:** hydrogel • **Moist:** calcium alginate, GFD*, foam • **Infected:** silver hydrogel, honey, PMD* with silver, cadexomer iodine, NaCl IG*, silver alginate	• Debridement only if needed to control odor, exudate, or infection. Use autolytic debridement methods, avoid surgical/sharp.
Exudate	• **None/Minimal Exudate:** contact layer, hydrogel, hydrocolloid, transparent film, composite dressing, petrolatum, petrolatum/3% Bismuth Tribromophenate (Xeroform™) gauze • **Moderate Exudate:** foam, calcium alginate, PMD* • **Heavy Exudate:** GFD* (Hydrofiber®), PMD* Max	• Protect periwound: apply skin barrier film or barrier cream • Avoid tape, if possible, use tubular netting, gauze roll, clothing to secure dressings
Infection	• **None/Minimal Exudate:** silver hydrogel, honey, PMD* with silver • **Moderate/Heavy Exudate:** silver foam, silver alginate, PMD* with silver, GFD* (Hydrofiber®) with silver, NaCl IG*, cadexomer iodine	• Anaerobic bacteria: use metronidazole to wound bed for ≤ 7 days; systemic metronidazole if wound is difficult to access; • Consider topical antimicrobials if multi-organism infection is suspected
Malodor	• **Cleansers*:** hypochlorous acid (Vashe®), sodium hypochlorite (Dakin's® 0.125%), acetic acid (0.25-0.5%) • **Dressings:** petrolatum/3% Bismuth Tribromophenate (Xeroform™) gauze, cadexomer iodine, honey, charcoal, silver, metronidazole (Flagyl®), essential oils (wintergreen or lavender) on dressing • **Environmental strategies:** kitty litter, vanilla extract, coffee grounds, dryer sheets placed in room	• Wound cleansing aids odor control. • Change dressing more often to manage odor. • Apply charcoal dressing and seal edges with tape to trap odors. • See infection above; topical or oral metronidazole
Dead Space	• Loosely fill dead space with the products listed above • Fistulas – See *page 104* for management of effluent	• Products are available in different forms, such as roping
Pruritus	• Hydrogel sheet covered with a transparent film • Hydrate skin by encouraging fluids and applying hydrophilic moisturizers, e.g., Lubriderm® or Cetaphil®	• Tumor stretching skin is a possible cause • Evaluate for contact dermatitis, hypersensitivity, or yeast dermatitis
Bleeding	• **Dressing strategies:** calcium alginate (silver alginate is not hemostatic), non-adherent dressing, or coagulants (gelatin sponge, thrombin) • **Topical/local strategies:** topical epinephrine or oxymetazoline, sclerosing agent (silver nitrate), antifibrinolytic agent (tranexamic acid), astringents (alum solution, sucralfate)	• Apply pressure for 10 to 15 minutes • Atraumatic removal of dressings – irrigate with normal saline to remove dressings. • Ask: Is the wound infected? Is patient on warfarin? Is transfusion appropriate? • Consider checking: platelet count, PT/INR, vitamin K deficiency
Support Surface	• Consider the need for a support surface only if a pressure injury is present.	• What was the causative injury?
Pain	**Nonpharmacological Interventions:** • **Procedural:** moisture-balanced, non-adherent, long-wear dressings; warm saline irrigation to remove dressings; time-outs; patient participation • **Complementary therapies:** music, relaxation, aromatherapy, visualization, meditation **Pharmacological Interventions:** • **Topical:** 2% lidocaine; EMLA® cream; morphine gel • **Systemic:** scheduled and pre-procedural opioid; tricyclic antidepressant; anticonvulsant	• Rule out infection or wound deterioration • Consider placing: hydrocolloid, foam, calcium alginate, PMD*, soft silicone, or hydrogel • EMLA® cream is applied to periwound tissue 60 minutes before the procedure • Morphine in hydrogel is only applied to open/inflamed wounds and must be compounded by a pharmacist.

***Cleansers:** Rinse wound bed with normal saline after using antiseptic cleanser to minimize toxic effects ‖**GFD:** Gelling fiber dressing
PMD: polymeric membrane dressing (PolyMem®)   **NaCl IG:** sodium chloride impregnated gauze (Mesalt®)

Treatment Algorithm for Malignant/Fungating Wounds

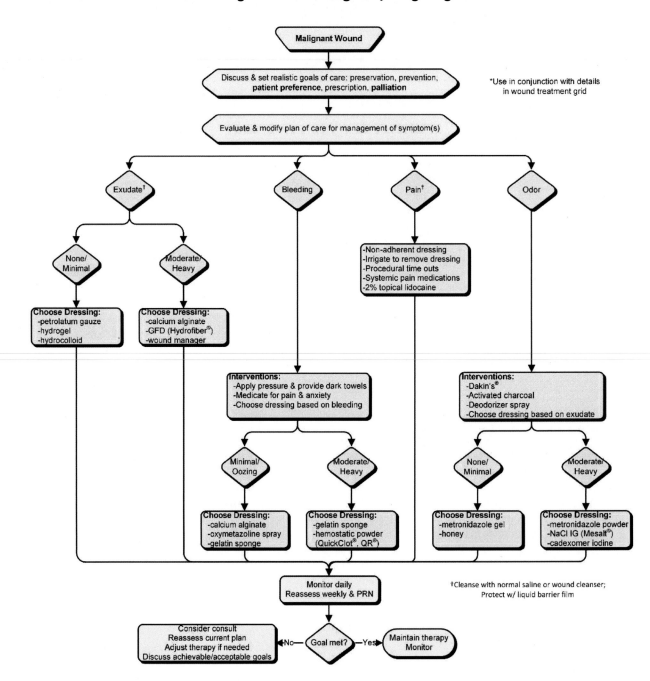

KEY POINTS

- A fungating or malignant wound is the manifestation of malignant cells that have infiltrated the skin and associated structures, such as blood and lymphatic vessels.
- Malignant wounds are a source of psychosocial distress, and wound care interventions should focus on relieving this distress.
- Non-adherent dressings are the intervention of choice for fungating wounds with patient-specific interventions to control odor, exudate, and bleeding.

CASE STUDY

The hospice nurse is admitting a 36-year-old female patient with a history of breast cancer. The patient presents with a fungating malignant wound to the right axilla measure 2.4 x 3.5 cm. The wound bed is 100% slough. The wound is distressing to the patient because of its significant odor and moderate exudate. Current treatment orders are honey with a composite dressing, changed daily. The nurse consults with the physician who provides the following wound care orders:

- Gently irrigate malignant wound of right axilla with normal saline. Pat periwound tissue dry. Apply metronidazole powder to wound bed daily x 7 days. After applying metronidazole, apply a composite charcoal dressing, and with a moisture-absorbing secondary dressing. Change dressing daily with the application of metronidazole and as needed if soiled.

The nurse demonstrates the application of the dressing, and the patient can return demonstrate the procedure. The nurse also assists the patient in placing kitty litter and an essential oil diffuser within her home. The nurse returns to the home the next week, and the patient notes a reduction in the wound odor. Moderate exudate is present. The physician discontinues the metronidazole. The physician continues the current dressing order to manage the exudate; however, the patient is instructed to change the dressing only when soiled or when strikethrough is present.

References

1. Bergstrom KJ. Assessment and management of fungating wounds. *J Wound Ostomy Continence Nurs.* 2011;38(1): 31-37.
2. Siu-ling EM, Wai-man CK. Management of malignant wound: nursing perspective. *HKSPM News.* 2004;2:11.
3. Wayne G. Impaired tissue integrity. September 13, 2016 https://nurseslabs.com/impaired-tissue-integrity/ Accessed October 12, 2017.
4. Seaman S. Management of malignant fungating wounds in advanced cancer. *Semin Oncol Nurs.* 2006;22(3):185-193.
5. Tilley C, Lipson J, Ramos M. Palliative wound care for malignant fungating wounds: holistic considerations at end-of-life. *Nurs Clin N Am.* 2016;51:513-531.
6. So-Shn Mak S, Lee MY, Cheung JSS, et al. Pressurised irrigation versus swabbing method in cleansing wounds healed by secondary intention. *Int J Nurs Stud.* 2015;52:88-101.
7. Popescu A, Sal Salcido R. Wound pain: a challenge for the patient and the wound care specialist. *Adv Skin Wound Care.* 2004;17(1):14-20.
8. Hebert GR. Palliative wound care: part 2. *Wound Care Advis* 2015;4(2).
9. Hopf HW, Shapshak D, Junkins S. Managing wound pain. In Bryant RA, Nix DP, eds. *Acute & Chronic Wounds: Current Management Concepts.* 4th ed. St Louis, MO:Elsevier/Mosby;2012:380-387
10. Tran QNH, Fancher T. Achieving analgesia for painful ulcers using topically applied morphine gel. *J Support Oncol.* 2007;5(6):289-293.

RADIATION DERMATITIS

GOALS

Within the confines of the patient's prognosis and in alignment with the wishes of the patient and family:

- Provide localized wound care with non-adherent dressings that maintain a moist wound bed
- Relieve distressing symptoms and promote quality of life

DEFINITIONS

Radiation dermatitis is a localized skin reaction due to the administration of radiation therapy. It usually occurs with therapeutic radiation rather than palliative radiation. Radiation dermatitis initially presents as mild **erythema**, which is a red rash on a previously radiated area. As it worsens, **dry desquamation** appears as pruritic, dry, flaking or peeling skin. In its most severe form, **moist desquamation** develops. Moist desquamation can range in severity from partial thickness tissue loss to life-threatening, full thickness skin ulcerations. Because of advances in therapeutic radiation therapy, the more severe form of moist desquamation is rare. Skin folds are at highest risk of experiencing radiation-induced skin changes because these areas usually receive the highest dose of radiation and can harbor bacteria.[1]

ASSESSMENT

Use the Radiation Therapy Oncology Group (RTOG) grading scale to assess the severity radiation dermatitis. Severity ranges from no noticeable skin changes (Grade 0) to death (Grade 5):[2]

> **Grade 0:** No observable skin changes
> **Grade 1:** Mild erythema, dry desquamation
> **Grade 2:** Bright erythema, edema, areas of moist desquamation in skin folds
> **Grade 3:** Moist desquamation outside of skin folds, pitting edema
> **Grade 4:** Full thickness skin ulcerations, hemorrhaging possible
> **Grade 5:** Death

PLAN OF CARE

Develop an individualized plan of care for the prevention and treatment of radiation dermatitis to guide the actions of all members of the interdisciplinary team. The care plan translates the data gained from the comprehensive assessment into a specific plan of action to prevent or manage radiation dermatitis. See Table 1 for potential care plans for radiation dermatitis.[2-4]

Table 1. Plan of Care for Radiation Dermatitis		
Nursing Diagnosis	**Related Factors**	**Interventions**
Risk for Impaired Skin Integrity • Patient has the potential for an alteration in skin integrity	• History of radiation therapy to the affected area • Friction, trauma • Altered nutritional status • Advanced age • Alcohol use, smoking • Obesity • Exposure to UV light • Comorbidities	• Assess skin, note areas of discoloration, texture, or temperature and any existing skin alterations • Encourage good skin care practices • Consult dietician, as needed • Avoid the use of adhesives • Maximize nutrition and hydration status • Assess skin alteration and determine etiology • Localized wound care, monitor daily
Impaired Skin Integrity • Partial thickness tissue loss		
Impaired Tissue Integrity • Full thickness tissue loss		

INTERVENTIONS

Prevention
All patients who have a history of radiation therapy or are currently receiving radiation therapy should follow general skin care practices to prevent radiation dermatitis:[3]

- Wash the radiated area daily with warm water and a mild soap. Use a mild shampoo if the radiated area is on the scalp. Pat dry with a soft towel. Avoid the use of wash clothes because of the risk of experiencing a friction injury.
- Although once discouraged, deodorants can be used.
- Avoid products with perfume, shaving with razors, waxing, or use of hair removal creams.
- Avoid direct exposure to heat or cold, direct sunlight, scratching or massaging of the skin, or the application of adhesives.
- Wear loose, breathable clothing.

Localized Wound Care
Treatment of radiation dermatitis depends on the level of severity. Maximum severity of the radiation dermatitis is seen 7 to 10 days after completion of treatment.[3] For mild erythema or dry desquamation, encourage the patient to apply an aqueous cream at least twice daily or more often, if needed. Avoid petroleum jelly products or products with irritants. Use 1% hydrocortisone to alleviate pruritus.[3]

If areas of moist desquamation with only partial thickness tissue loss are present, the principles of moist wound healing apply. Non-adherent foam dressings, such as Mepilex®, PolyMem®, or Allevyn®, will manage exudate while minimizing pain. Yellow to green exudate is normal. Do not remove this exudate unless it is excessive. Silver dressings are useful if an infection is present. Continue to use aqueous creams in areas of intact, erythematous skin or areas of dry desquamation. Use topical steroids for pruritus but only apply to areas of intact skin.[3] If full thickness tissue loss is present, with or without hemorrhage, consult a wound specialist to rule out the need for debridement or skin grafting, if in alignment with the goals and wishes of the patient.[3] Otherwise, use the above-mentioned dressings for autolytic debridement and moisture management. The following algorithm and treatment grid outline the management of radiation dermatitis.

WOUND TREATMENT GRID: Radiation Dermatitis[3,5]		
Wound Need	**Intervention**	**Comments**
Cleanse	• **Clean wound bed:** pour normal saline or wound cleanser • Normal saline soaks to loosen crusting	• Refrain from removing the yellow to green exudate unless excessive
Debridement	• **Dry:** hydrogel, PMD* • **Moist:** non-adherent foam (PMD*, Allevyn®, Mepilex®) • **Infected:** silver hydrogel, silver foam, PMD* with silver	• Emergent consult if necrotic tissue is present • Moisten PMD* with saline if wound bed is dry
Exudate	• **Dry Desquamation:** aqueous cream (e.g., Aquaphor®) at least two times daily • **Moist Desquamation:** hydrogel, calcium alginate, non-adherent foam (PMD*, Allevyn®, Mepilex®)	• Moisten PMD* with saline in a dry wound bed • Avoid tape, use tubular netting or gauze roll to secure dressings
Infection	• **None/Minimal Exudate:** honey, silver hydrogel • **Moderate Exudate/Heavy Exudate:** silver non-adherent foam (PMD* with silver), honey alginate	• Uncommon with these wounds • Limit the use of topical antibiotics*
Malodor	• **Cleansers*:** hypochlorous acid (Vashe®) • **Dressings:** honey, charcoal, metronidazole (Flagyl®) to wound bed, essential oils (wintergreen or lavender) on dressing • **Environmental strategies:** kitty litter, vanilla extract, coffee grounds, dryer sheets placed in room	• Rule out infection • Wound cleansing aids odor control • Change dressing more often to manage odor
Dead Space	• Rare unless severe reaction • Loosely fill dead space with the products listed above	• Products are available in different forms, such as roping
Pruritus	• 1% hydrocortisone cream to intact skin only • Normal saline compresses • Cooled hydrogel sheets	• Evaluate for contact dermatitis, hypersensitivity, or yeast dermatitis
Bleeding	• **Dressing strategies:** calcium alginate (silver alginate is not hemostatic), non-adherent dressings, or coagulants (gelatin sponge, thrombin) • **Topical/local strategies:** sclerosing agent (silver nitrate), antifibrinolytic agent (tranexamic acid), astringents (alum solution, sucralfate), vasoconstrictive agents [topical oxymetazoline (Afrin®), topical epinephrine]	• Atraumatic removal of dressings – irrigate with normal saline to remove dressings. • Ask: Is the wound infected? Is patient on warfarin? Is transfusion appropriate? • Consider checking: platelet count, PT/INR, vitamin K deficiency • Use topical vasoconstrictors only when bleeding is minimal, oozing, or seeping
Support Surface	• Consider the need for a support surface only if a pressure injury is present.	• What was the causative injury?
Pain	**Nonpharmacological Interventions:** • **Procedural:** moisture-balanced, non-adherent, long-wear dressings; warm saline irrigation to remove dressings; time-outs; patient participation • **Complementary therapies:** music, relaxation, aromatherapy, visualization, meditation **Pharmacological Interventions:** • **Systemic:** scheduled and pre-procedural opioid; tricyclic antidepressant; anticonvulsant	• Rule out infection or wound deterioration • Consider placing: foam, PMD*, soft silicone, or hydrogel

*Cleansers: Rinse wound bed with normal saline after using antiseptic cleanser to minimize toxic effects
PMD: polymeric membrane dressing (PolyMem®)
Topical Antibiotics: Use of a topical antibiotic is NOT recommended due to the potential for adverse reactions and antimicrobial resistance

Treatment Algorithm for Radiation Dermatitis

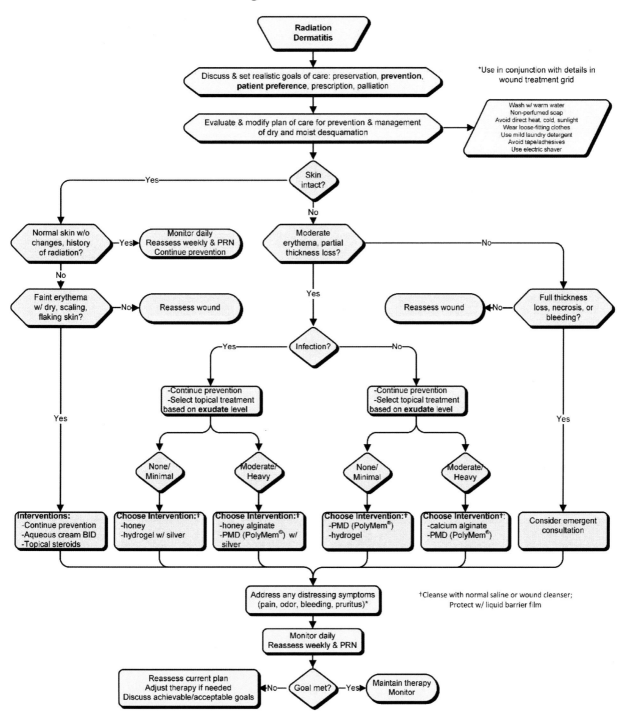

KEY POINTS

- Radiation dermatitis is a localized skin reaction due to the administration of radiation therapy.
- Dry desquamation appears as pruritic, dry, flaking, or peeling skin.
- Moist desquamation appears as partial thickness tissue loss within the folds of the skin in mild cases but can also present as extensive, full thickness tissue loss in severe cases.
- Grade radiation dermatitis on a scale from 0 to 5, with 0 being the absence of symptoms and 5 implying that the patient has died as a result of the injury.
- Apply aqueous cream at least twice daily in dry desquamation.
- Use non-adherent dressings for moist desquamation.

CASE STUDY

The hospice nurse is admitting a 63-year-old female patient with a history of lung cancer. The patient just completed a round of chemotherapy and radiation without success one week ago. The patient complains of pruritus and erythema to the left anterior chest wall. The nurse assesses the area and suspects radiation dermatitis, Grade 1. The nurse recommends applying an aqueous cream at least twice daily to the area. Upon physician notification of the presence of radiation dermatitis and the patient's complaint of pruritus, an order is also placed for 1% hydrocortisone cream to be applied to the affected area twice daily for up to seven days, discontinue after 24 hours if no response to treatment. The nurse reviews the orders with the patient who verbalizes understanding. The nurse also educates the patient that because the last radiation treatment was completed one week ago, this is most likely the maximum severity of the reaction, and improvement should be seen with these interventions.

References
1. Salvo N, Barnes E, van Draanen J, et al. Prophylaxis and management of acute radiation-induced skin reactions: a systematic review of the literature. *Curr Oncol*. 2010;17(4):94-112.
2. Trueman E. Management of radiotherapy-induced skin reactions. *Int J of Palliat Nurs*. 2015;21(4):187-192.
3. Trueman E, Princess Royal Radiotherapy Review Team. *Managing Radiotherapy Induced Skin Reactions: A Toolkit for Healthcare professionals*. Leeds, UK: St James's Institute of Oncology; 2011 https://www.sor.org/system/files/news_story/201204/ltht-managingradiotherapyinducedskinreactions-oct2011.pdf. Accessed October 19, 2017.
4. Vera M. Four dermatitis care plans. January 25, 2012 https://nurseslabs.com/dermatitis-nursing-care-plans/. Accessed October 13, 2017.
5. Hopf HW, Shapshak D, Junkins S. Managing wound pain. In Bryant RA, Nix DP, eds. *Acute & Chronic Wounds: Current Management Concepts.* 4th ed. St Louis, MO:Elsevier/Mosby;2012:380-387.

NUTRITION

GOALS

Within the confines of the patient's prognosis and in alignment with the wishes of the patient and family:

- Maximize nutritional status to promote wound healing if appropriate and in alignment with the wishes and goals of the patient and caregiver
- Relieve distressing symptoms contributing to the impaired nutritional status and promote quality of life

DEFINITIONS

Wound healing is an intricate process that is dependent upon the availability of nutritional resources for success. Any decline in nutritional status increases the risk of developing a wound and delays or halts wound healing. Maximizing the nutritional status of any patient that demonstrates signs or symptoms of a nutritional decline is generally considered the standard of care.[1] Unfortunately, at the end of life, these interventions may be futile. The perception that patients who show a nutritional decline are only malnourished is erroneous. **Malnutrition** develops when the body lacks the essential protein and nutrients needed to flourish. The most advanced form of malnutrition, **starvation**, is painful and can lead to death. Malnutrition is reversible with nutritional interventions; however, in advanced disease and at the end of life, the observed nutritional decline can be much more complicated than merely a lack of essential nutrients. Instead, these patients may suffer from cachexia. **Cachexia** is muscle wasting due to advanced disease. Cachexia is a metabolic syndrome, and, as a result, nutritional interventions alone do not improve the patient's outcome. These patients may also demonstrate **anorexia** (loss of appetite).[2] Although the loss of appetite and involuntary weight loss can be distressing to the family, it is a natural part of the dying process. Maximizing nutritional status to enhance wound healing at the end of life is often not appropriate. Only a comprehensive nutritional assessment and a discussion of realistic and desired goals of care will yield the determination of the appropriateness of nutritional interventions.

ASSESSMENT

Complete a nutritional screening upon admission and with any change in condition to identify the need for a comprehensive nutritional assessment. Conduct the screening with a valid and reliable tool (see page 119 for sample nutritional assessments). If a nutritional assessment is warranted, a registered dietician is an ideal clinician to complete the assessment. If appropriate, also consult a dietician for any patient with a new or existing pressure injury.[3]

Typical components of a nutritional screening and assessment include:[3,4]

- An accurate weight to identify significant weight loss and calculate body mass index (BMI). Significant weight loss is designated by a loss of 5% or more in 30 days or 10% or more in 180 days. A BMI less than 18.5 can indicate malnutrition.
- Identification of barriers to maintaining nutritional status, such as the inability to feed self, difficulty swallowing, loss of appetite, nausea/vomiting, mouth pain, or cognitive decline.
- Fluid, calorie, and protein intake counts and current requirements.
- A review of any available laboratory studies, such as albumin, prealbumin, transferrin, retinol-binding protein, C-reactive protein, total lymphocyte count, and serum total cholesterol. Note that the albumin level is affected by other factors, such as inflammation and hydration status, and is not used to determine the need for protein supplementation.

Ultimately, the information gained from the nutritional screening and assessment will assist in developing a plan of care that maximizes the nutrition of the patient if appropriate and in alignment with the goals and wishes of the patient and caregiver.[3]

PLAN OF CARE

Develop an individualized plan of care for the management of nutritional decline to guide the actions of all members of the interdisciplinary team. The care plan translates the data gained from completion of the nutritional screening and assessment into a specific plan of action to maximize nutrition based on the wishes and goals of the patient and/or caregiver. Table 1 reviews potential care plans for nutrition:[5]

Table 1. Care Plans for Nutrition[5]		
Nursing Diagnosis	Related Factors	Interventions
Imbalanced Nutrition: Less Than Body Requirements • Nutrient intake is insufficient to support the metabolic needs of the patient.	• Inability to consume, digest, or absorb foods • Advanced disease processes causing increased nutrient needs • Loss of appetite or lack of desire to eat	• Dietician referral, as appropriate. • Identify realistic and achievable goals of care. • Ensure meal environment is pleasant. • Position the patient to maximize swallowing. • Oral care before and after meals and as needed. • Provide smaller, more frequent meals throughout the day. • Provide the largest meal of the day at the time the patient is most hungry, no matter what time of day that is. • Liberalized diet. • Nutritional supplements or vitamins if appropriate and in alignment with patient's goals of care.

INTERVENTIONS

Implement nutritional interventions to maximize wound healing if compatible with the patient's condition and wishes, including supplements, medications, and nonpharmacological interventions.[3,6] Note that some appetite stimulant medications also hinder wound healing (e.g., corticosteroids, such as prednisone or dexamethasone) or cause adverse effects for patients [e.g., DVT risk with megestrol (Megace®);

sedation and xerostomia with mirtazapine (Remeron®)].[7] Only recommend vitamin C and zinc for patients with a documented nutritional deficiency.[1] Recommend the following approaches for the alert patient able to tolerate food and drink safely:[1,6,8-10]

- Small, frequent meals of the patient's desired food or drink
- Relaxed dietary restrictions
- Supplements for patients with protein, vitamin, or mineral deficiencies
- Water or other fluids within easy reach, encouraging small, frequent sips
- Easy to swallow foods, such as gelatin, pudding, ice cream, popsicles, or soup
- High-protein diet. Add protein powder to foods, such as pudding, soups, or milkshakes, or choose foods high in protein.
- Prevention and management oral mucositis and xerostomia

Review the overall goals and wishes of the patient, family, and care team before implementing enteral or parenteral nutrition.[8] Only consider enteral tube feedings or parenteral nutrition if they are in line with the patient's wishes and the treatment of malnutrition will increase the possibility of wound healing.[11,12] Support for the use of enteral nutrition to prevent or heal pressure injuries is conflicting. In some instances, the use of a PEG tube increases the risk of developing a pressure injury, particularly in nursing home patients with advanced dementia. Tube feeding necessitates the elevation of the head of the bed (HOB) increasing pressure, shear, and friction. Use of feeding tubes does not improve survival or prevent aspiration pneumonia. Use of feeding tubes also decreases human interaction because solitary feedings in a patient room replaces meals with other individuals or family members.[13]

KEY POINTS

- Malnutrition develops when the body lacks the essential protein and energy needed to flourish. It is reversible through nutritional interventions.
- Cachexia is muscle wasting due to advanced disease. It cannot be reversed through nutritional interventions.
- Complete a nutritional screening upon admission and with any change in condition to identify the need for a comprehensive nutritional assessment.
- Implement nutritional interventions to maximize wound healing if compatible with the patient's condition and wishes.
- Critically review the overall goals and wishes of the patient, family, and care team before implementing enteral or parenteral nutrition.

References

1. Wild T, Rahbarnia A, Kellner M, et al. Basics in nutrition and wound healing. *Nutrition.* 2010; 26:862-866.
2. Kroustos KR. Anorexia and cachexia. In: Protus BM, Kimbrel J, Grauer P, eds. *Palliative Care Consultant: A Reference Guide for Palliative Care.* Montgomery, AL: HospiScript, a Catamaran Company; 2015:23-27.
3. National Pressure Ulcer Advisory Panel (NPUAP), European Pressure Ulcer Advisory Panel (EPUAP) and Pan Pacific Pressure Injury Alliance. Prevention and Treatment of Pressure Ulcers: Quick Reference Guide. Emily Haesler (Ed.). Cambridge Media: Osborne Park, Western Australia; 2014.
4. Collins N. Using laboratory data to evaluate nutritional status. *Ostomy Wound Manage.* March 2010. http://www.o-wm.com/files/owm/pdfs/Nutrition411.2_Mar2010.pdf. Accessed October 12, 2017.
5. Wayne, G. Imbalanced nutrition: less than body requirements. August 25, 2016. https://nurseslabs.com/imbalanced-nutrition-less-body-requirements/ Accessed October 12, 2017.

6. Posthauer ME. Palliative care challenges: offering supportive nutritional care at end of life. May 1, 2012 http://www.woundsource.com/blog/palliative-care-challenges-offering-supportive-nutritional-care-end-life Accessed October 12, 2017.
7. Lexi-Drugs Online. Lexicomp. Wolters Kluwer; Hudson, OH. Accessed April 16, 2018.
8. Lyder CH, Ayello EA. Pressure ulcers: a patient safety issue. In: Hughes R. ed. *Patient Safety and Quality: An Evidence-Based Handbook for Nurses*. AHRQ Pub No. 08-0043. Rockville, MD; Agency for Healthcare Research and Quality; 2008:i276-i299. https://www.ncbi.nlm.nih.gov/books/NBK2650/. Accessed October 12, 2017.
9. O'Brien CP. Management of stomatitis. *Can Fam Physician*. 2009;55:891-892.
10. Wiseman M. The treatment of oral problems in the palliative patient. *J Can Dent Assoc.* 2006;72(5):453-458.
11. Stotts N. Nutritional assessment and support. In Bryant RA, Nix DP, eds. *Acute & Chronic Wounds: Current Management Concepts.* 4th ed. St Louis, MO:Elsevier/Mosby;2012:388-399.
12. Alvarez OM, Kalinski C, Nusbaum J, et al. Incorporating wound healing strategies to improve palliation (symptom management) in patients with chronic wounds. *J Palliat Med.* 2007;10(5):1161-1189.
13. Teno J, Gozalo P, Mitchell SL, et al. Feeding tubes and the prevention or healing of pressure ulcers. *Arch Intern Med.* 2012;172(9):697-701.

SPECIAL TOPICS

GOALS

- Discuss the pathophysiology and local wound care treatment of calciphylaxis, Marjolin's ulcers, lymphedema, and enterocutaneous fistulas
- Identify peristomal skin complications and subsequent treatment options
- Identify common skin rashes and appropriate interventions to relieve distressing symptoms

CALCIPHYLAXIS

Calciphylaxis is the calcification of small vessels, which usually presents as painful mottling of the skin that deteriorates to necrosis. The lesions appear on areas with the greatest amount of subcutaneous fat, such as the upper thighs, abdomen, or buttocks; however, calciphylaxis can affect internal organs, such the heart or digestive system. Calciphylaxis is most common in patients with chronic renal failure and dialysis, but can occur in other disease processes, such as multiple myeloma, cirrhosis, or rheumatoid arthritis.[1]

Calciphylaxis signals a poor prognosis, with survival estimates less than 1 year.[2] Typical management of the disease requires administration of medications, surgical debridement of necrotic tissue, more frequent dialysis, diet modification, and surgical removal of the parathyroid gland. For the palliative care patient, this intensive treatment may not be in alignment with the patient's wishes. Therefore, at the end of life, the onset of calciphylaxis should trigger a conversation with the patient and family regarding prognosis and goals of care. If the patient is currently receiving dialysis, discuss cessation of dialysis.

The necrotic lesions of calciphylaxis are painful and odorous. Do not attempt debridement of the necrotic tissue if dry, stable, non-infected eschar is present. Instead, paint the wound with povidone-iodine and leave it open to air. If the eschar is unstable and or if an infection is present, consider consulting a wound specialist for recommendations [e.g., surgical debridement or cautious debridement with collagenase (Santyl®)]. After debridement, select dressings to maintain a moist wound bed. Use odor absorbing dressings (e.g., charcoal) to prevent patient embarrassment. Extend the wear time of the dressing to avoid frequent and painful dressing changes.[1,3]

Pain is the most distressing symptom of calciphylaxis, potentially from both ischemic tissue and a neuropathic component. Unfortunately, pain can be refractory to opioids and disproportionate to the level of tissue damage observed. Additionally, the compromised renal state of the patient increases risk for opioid toxicity. The limited data available regarding management of this refractory pain suggests the concurrent use of an opioid, benzodiazepine, and gabapentin or pregabalin provides the best pain relief for these patients. If pain is refractory, consider adding subcutaneous ketamine to the regimen.[2,3]

References
1. Magro CM, Simman R, Jackson S. Calciphylaxis: a review. *J Am Coll Clin Wound Spec.* 2010;2(4):66-72.
2. Nigwekar S, Thadhani R, Bradenburg V. Calciphylaxis. *N Engl J Med.* 2018;378:1704-1714.
3. Polizzotto MN, Bryan T, Ashby M, Martin P. Symptomatic management of calciphylaxis. *J Pain Symptom Manage.* 2006;32(2):186-190.

MARJOLIN'S ULCERS

Marjolin's ulcers reflect malignant changes in scar tissue or the wound bed of a chronic ulceration. Punch biopsy of the lesion reveals squamous cell carcinoma. They are usually found on the lower extremities and are most frequently associated with burn scars, but they can also occur with pressure injuries, venous ulcers, or scars from lupus, vaccinations, or radiation. The typical presentation of a Marjolin's ulcer is an indurated nodule with ulceration at a scar site; however, they can also appear flat with indurated, elevated margins. In a chronic wound, evidence of malignancy includes pain, bleeding, increase in size, hypergranulation tissue, epibole, foul-smelling and purulent drainage, or any wound present greater than three months. Malignant wounds, including Marjolin's ulcers, are considered non-healing wounds requiring a palliative care focus; rule out a Marjolin's ulcer in any non-healing wound.[1,2]

Marjolin's ulcers are slow to metastasize. The scar tissue, which is poorly vascularized, slows metastasis. Once the cancerous cells reach vascularized tissue, metastasis is possible, and disease progression is rapid. Marjolin's ulcers usually metastasize to the lymph nodes, brain, liver, lungs, or kidneys.[1]

Treatment of a Marjolin's ulcer involves tumor resection, lymph node dissection, or amputation. Re-occurrence is possible. At the end of life, the management of Marjolin's ulcers requires the use of topical dressings to control the distressing symptoms of the tumors, whether that is pain, odor, bleeding, or exudate. Monitor for symptoms of metastasis and address symptoms as they occur.[1]

References
1. Pekarek B, Buck S, Osher L. A comparison review on Marjolin's ulcers: diagnosis and treatment. *J Am Col Certif Wound Spec*. 2011;3(3):60-64.
2. Maida V, Ennis M, Kuziemsky C, Trozzolo L. Symptoms associated with malignant wounds: a prospective case series. J Pain Symptom Manage 2009; 37(2):206-211.

LYMPHEDEMA

Lymphedema is the result of a defect of the lymphatic system leading to a buildup of interstitial fluid either due to an anomaly present at birth or as a result of cancer treatment, burns, or trauma. This interstitial fluid is high in protein and cellular debris and results in swelling of the affected tissues.[1,2] Lymphedema is a progressive disease and, without treatment, will result in chronic inflammation, skin changes, recurrent infection (cellulitis or abscess), and skin ulcerations. These ulcerations can range in size from a small, localized lesion to circumferential and can become chronic unless the underlying disease process can be resolved. Localized wound care focuses on managing exudate, which is usually heavy, while treating the underlying disease process.[1-3]

The gold standard of treatment for lymphedema is Complete Decongestive Therapy (CDT). There are five components to CDT:[1-4]

- Manual lymph drainage: Method of lightly touching the skin to cause the movement of interstitial fluid out of the tissue and into the lymphatic system. A specially trained clinician performs manual lymph drainage. Simple lymphatic drainage, on the other hand, is performed by the patient to maintain the fluid reduction achieved with manual lymph drainage.

- Short-stretch compression bandaging: Provides firm support for muscles to push against to facilitate lymphatic fluid movement. Note that ace bandages are considered long-stretch bandages and are not appropriate for lymphedema compression.
- Lymphatic exercises: Muscle contraction results in the flow of lymph through the lymphatic system.
- Preventive skin care: Wash daily with a pH balanced skin cleanser followed by application of a moisturizer. Hyperkeratotic skin is common with lymphedema and removal of the buildup is recommended to allow penetration of moisturizers. A debriding mitt can be used to assist in the gentle removal of the hyperkeratotic buildup.
- Patient education regarding management and compression.

CDT consists of two phases: the initial reduction phase of interstitial fluid (phase 1) and the maintenance phase (phase 2). Phase 1 of CDT is performed daily for up to eight weeks or until the maximum fluid volume reduction is reached. Upon completion, the patient moves to phase 2 to maintain fluid reduction through self-care activities, including simple lymphatic drainage, lymphatic exercises, preventive skin care regimen, and application of compression bandages or compression garments.[1-4]

References

1. National Lymphedema Network (NLN) Advisory Committee. Position statement of the National Lymphedema Network. February 2011. https://www.lymphnet.org/pdfDocs/nlntreatment.pdf Accessed July 24, 2017.
2. Kercher K, Fleisher A, Yosipovitch G. Lower extremity lymphedema. Update: pathophysiology, diagnosis, and treatment guidelines. *J Am Acad Dermatol.* 2008;59(2):324-331.
3. Karnasula VM. Management of ulcers in lymphoedematous limbs. *Indian J Plast Surg.* 2012;45(2):261-265.
4. Nowicki J, Siviour A. Best practice skin care management in lymphedema. *Wound Practice and Research.* 2013;21(2):61-65.

ENTEROCUTANEOUS FISTULAS

An enterocutaneous fistula is an opening between a part of the gastrointestinal tract (stomach, small intestine, or large intestine) and the skin. Fistulas are the result of surgery or can occur spontaneously secondary to trauma, inflammatory bowel disease, cancer, diverticulitis, or radiation. Classify enterocutaneous fistulas as simple or complex and by the volume of output:[1,2]

- Simple fistulas are short with a direct tract between the skin and the affected portion of the gastrointestinal tract.
- Complex fistulas can terminate within a wound, involve other adjacent organs, or contain an abscess.
- High-output fistulas generate more than 500 mL of effluent in a 24 hour period.
- Low-output fistulas generate less than 200 mL of effluent in a 24 hour period.

Complications of enterocutaneous fistulas include malnutrition, imbalances of fluid and electrolytes, skin damage from the corrosive effluent, pain, odor, sepsis, and death. Effective management of an enterocutaneous fistula at the end of life involves protection of the skin, containment of the effluent, odor control, and support of the patient.[1,2] Table 1 provides guidance on management of fistula effluent to protect the surrounding skin.

Table 1. Topical Management of the Enterocutaneous Fistula Effluent[1,2]		
• **Effluent volume < 100 mL/24 hours?** • **Dressing change required < every 4 hours?**	Odor Absent	• Topical dressings, such as gauze, alginate, foam, or gelling fiber dressings (Hydrofiber®) • Barrier creams, liquid barrier film, or ostomy rings, pastes, or powders to protect surrounding skin
	Odor Present	• Charcoal dressings, ostomy deodorants • Increase frequency of dressing changes • Fistula pouches, wound management system, ostomy pouching systems, either one piece or two piece
• **Effluent volume > 100 mL/24 hours?** • **Dressing change required > every 4 hours?**	Odor Absent	• Fistula pouches, wound management system, ostomy pouching system, either one piece or two piece
	Odor Present	• Ostomy deodorants • Fistula pouches, wound management system, ostomy pouching system, either one piece or two piece
• **Erosion of surrounding skin?**		• Ulcerated areas – apply alginate, gelling fiber dressings (Hydrofiber®), or hydrocolloid to the wound bed before applying appliance • Inflamed or denuded areas – use crusting technique (see page 59)

References

1. Wound Ostomy and Continence Nurses Society®. The Wound, Ostomy and Continence Nurses Society™ (WOCN®) support of Medicare coverage for enterocutaneous fistulas. http://c.ymcdn.com/sites/www.wocn.org/resource/resmgr/AdvocacyPolicy/Support_of_Medicare_Coverage. pdf. Approved March 2015. Accessed July 26, 2017.
2. McNaughton, V. Canadian Association for Enterostomal Therapy ECF Best Practice Recommendations Panel. Summary of best practice recommendations for management of enterocutaneous fistulae from the Canadian Association for Enterostomal Therapy ECF Best Practice Recommendations Panel. *J Wound Ostomy Continence Nurs.* 2010;37(2):173-184.

CARE OF THE STOMA

A stoma is the visible part of the gastrointestinal tract brought through the abdominal wall after an ostomy procedure. Common indications for performing an ostomy include cancer, ulcerative colitis, Crohn's disease, extensive wounds, or trauma. The effluent of a stoma will be either urine or stool. The consistency of the stool varies based upon the location of the ostomy. Numerous peristomal skin complications can occur, and management of these complications is imperative to the relief of distressing symptoms at the end of life.[1-4] Routinely assess peristomal skin for signs of trauma from ostomy equipment, infection, irritants such as feces, urine, or ostomy effluent, allergens, other skin syndromes.[5] Table 2 provides general guidance for managing peristomal complications.

Table 2. Treatment of Peristomal Skin Complications[1-5]

Peristomal Skin Complication	Treatment

Mechanical Trauma
• Pressure injury – related to the use of convex pouches or too tight of an ostomy belt
• Shear/friction – harsh removal of appliance or abrasive cleaning
	• Pressure injury – relieve the pressure
	   o Evaluate necessity for convex system
	   o Secure belt snugly but not excessively tight
	• Shear/friction
	   o Teach patient/caregiver to gently remove pouch and provide gentle cleansing
	   o Refrain from using extra adhesives (e.g., cement)
	   o Remove pouch system in direction of hair growth
	• Ulcerated areas – apply calcium alginate, gelling fiber dressing (Hydrofiber®), or hydrocolloid to the wound bed before applying appliance
	• Denuded areas – use crusting technique (see page 59)

Infection – Bacterial or Fungal
• Candidiasis – bright red rash related to a warm, moist environment created by the pouching system
• Folliculitis – infection of hair follicles, usually from incorrect shaving of the area or from traumatic removal of the pouching system
	• Candidiasis
	   o Antifungal powder
	   o Change appliance with each application of powder
	• Folliculitis
	   o Shave hair in the direction of hair growth using an electric razor
	   o Gentle removal of pouching system
	   o Oral antibiotic
	• Crusting technique may be necessary to assist with pouch adherence (see page 59)

Chemical Irritants
• Contact dermatitis – related to effluent
• Hyperplasia – appears as discolored papules or nodules, usually related to prolonged exposure to urine or stool
• Alkaline encrustations – crystal formations, usually from exposure to alkaline urine, urinary tract infections, concentrated urine, or kidney stones
	• See page 104 for management of effluent-related skin damage
	• Hyperplasia
	   o Correctly fit pouching system
	   o Convex pouch if stoma is flush or retracted
	• Alkaline encrustations related to urostomy
	   o Vinegar soaks
	   o Rule out infection and presence of kidney stones

Diseases
• Pyoderma gangrenosum – inflammatory autoimmune disease, starts as pustules and leads to painful ulcerations of the skin. Treatments are usually immunosuppressant or anti-inflammatory medications
	• Topical treatment
	   o Triamcinolone 40 mg/mL injected into ulcer edge
	   o Topical tacrolimus
	• Systemic treatment
	   o Corticosteroids
	   o Cyclosporine

Allergens
• Allergic contact dermatitis – rash that mirrors the shape of the offending agent, usually related to the use of pouching system or other stoma products
• Granulomas – often related to retained suture fragments or from injury from the pouching system
	• Allergic contact dermatitis
	   o Identify offending agent and discontinue use
	   o Conduct a patch test before using a new product
	• Granulomas
	   o Silver nitrate up to three times per week
	   o Stoma paste at the site to prevent injury from the pouching system

References

1. Wound Care Education Institute. It's complicated! Ostomy patients and peristomal skin. March 18, 2016. https://blog.wcei.net/2016/03/its-complicated-ostomy-patients-and-peristomal-skin Accessed May 30, 2017.
2. Jordan R, Christian M. Understanding peristomal skin complications. Wound Care Advisor. 2013;2(3):2 https://woundcareadvisor.com/understanding-periostomal-skin-complications_vol2_no3/ Accessed May 30, 2017.
3. Brooklyn T, Dunnill G, Probert C. Diagnosis and treatment of pyoderma gangrenosum. *BMJ*. 2006;333(7560):181-184.

4. Johnson T. Problematic stomas...stoma granulomas. Colostomy Association Web site. http://www.colostomyassociation.org.uk/_assets/File/pdf/Articles%20from%20previous%20Tidings/Granulo mas.pdf. Accessed May 31, 2017.
5. Woo K, Sibbald G, Ayello E, Coutts P, Garde D. Peristomal skin complications and management. *Adv Skin Wound Care* 2009;22(11):522-532

IDENTIFICATION OF COMMON SKIN RASHES

Skin rashes are challenging to diagnose and treat. Begin a skin rash evaluation with a comprehensive history and physical assessment. Obtain a complete medication list, inquire about sun exposure, discuss recent travel, identify associated signs and symptoms, such as fever, and obtain information regarding products used within the home, including soaps, detergents, solvents, or cleaning solutions.[1] Describe the lesion using the descriptors provided in the Table 3.[1-2] After correctly describing the lesion and obtaining a thorough patient history, use Table 4 to identify the type of skin lesion and the preferred method of treatment.

Table 3. Skin Rash Descriptors[1-2]		
Character Descriptor		**Definition**
Primary Skin Lesions		**Present at the initial onset of the skin condition**
Flat, non-palpable discoloration of the skin	Macule	A flat mark; circular area of color (brown, tan, red, white); <1 cm
	Patch	A flat mark; circular area of color (brown, tan, red, white); >1 cm
Elevated, palpable solid masses	Nodule	Elevated; firm, circular, palpable; typically >1 cm in diameter
	Papule	Superficial, elevated; palpable, firm, circular lesion; <1 cm
	Plaque	Superficial, elevated, flat-topped; >1 cm
	Wheal	Elevated; edematous, transient
Elevated, palpable, fluid-filled masses	Vesicle	Elevated; superficial, circular, fluid-filled blister; <1 cm
	Bulla	Elevated; superficial, circular, fluid-filled blister; >1 cm
	Pustule	Elevated; superficial, pus-filled blister; variable sizes
Secondary Skin Lesions		**Result of changes over time (disease progression, scratching) or treatments**
Scale		Epidermal thickening; flaky exfoliation, dry or oily, silver, white, or tan
Crust		Slightly elevated; dried serum or exudate on the skin
Excoriation		Superficial loss of epidermis (linear area usually due to scratching)
Lichenification		Rough, thickened epidermis; exaggeration of normal skim markings secondary to scratching

Table 4. Empiric Treatment by Type of Rash[1-15]

Rash	Distinguishing Characteristics	Etiology	Empiric Treatment
Bullous Pemphigoid[1,3]	• Bulla present on the trunk and areas of skin flexure (e.g., abdomen, axilla, upper thighs), age >70	• Autoimmune disease affecting cohesion of dermis and epidermis	• Topical clobetasol propionate 0.05% (40 grams per day) • Oral prednisolone (0.5-1 mg/kg/day)
Bed Bugs[4,5]	• Linear groups of 3 bites with pruritus • Appears as macular lesions that become wheals (5 cm in diameter); pruritic, erythematous papules	• Bites of *Cimex lectularius* and *Cimex hemipterus*	• Low-potency topical corticosteroids (hydrocortisone 0.1% cream) for a maximum of 2 weeks • Antihistamines (loratadine, cetirizine) • Treat the environment
Cutaneous Candidiasis[6]	• Areas of erythema with satellite papules and pustules, usually in the folds of the skin, with or without pruritus, odor, or pain	• Overgrowth of *Candida* in warm, moist environments, may spread across a large area	• Topical antifungals applied BID • Oral fluconazole 100-200 mg daily x 7 days if resistant to topicals • Good personal hygiene • Rule out irritant contact dermatitis
Cellulitis[7]	• Unilateral, red, swollen area that is warm and tender to touch; may appear tight and shiny; will spread rapidly	• Bacterial infection of the skin and underlying soft tissues	• Antibiotics: cephalexin, amoxicillin-clavulanic acid; MRSA: clindamycin, doxycycline, sulfamethoxazole-trimethoprim • Elevate affected extremity
Allergic Contact Dermatitis[8,9]	• Erythematous rash in area exposed to the offending agent, with or without pruritus, vesicles, or bullae	• Repeated exposure to an allergen (latex, metals, plants, dyes, etc.) • Occurs within 12-72 hours of exposure	• Cool moist compresses • Topical or oral steroids • Calamine lotion • Limit exposure to offending agent
Irritant Contact Dermatitis[8,9]	• Tender, red, scaly rash with poorly defined borders; maceration if moisture is causative agent	• Repeated exposure to an irritant (water, soap, urine/stool, etc.)	• Emollients, topical/oral steroids • Limit exposure to offending agent • If related to moisture, treat based on etiology (see *MASD* page 57)
Drug Rash[10]	• Erythema, wheals, urticaria (hives), maculopapular rash, skin peeling, or blistering of mucous membranes	• Allergic or nonallergic skin reaction due to a medication side effect, usually within 1-2 weeks of initiating a mediation	• Medication review • Discontinue offending drug • Antihistamines • Oral steroids • May vary based on specific reaction
Eczema[11] **(Atopic Dermatitis)**	• Chronic dry, red, pruritic skin, especially on the hands, feet, chest, eyelids, knees, or elbows	• Genetic variation that reduces the skin's ability to protect against allergens and irritants	• Emollients • Topical or oral steroids
Folliculitis[12]	• Tender, red pustules, usually on the face, chest, back, buttocks, or legs with or without pruritus	• Inflammation of hair follicles due to bacterial or fungal infection, shaving, or blockage	• Topical or oral antibiotics, antifungals, antibacterial soap • Electric razor, shaving cream • Warm compresses
Scabies[13]	• Red, intensely pruritic papular rash usually of the webs of fingers, wrists, elbows, knees, and waist	• *Sarcoptes scabiei* burrows in to the skin	• Permethrin or lindane topically • Ivermectin orally • Diphenhydramine for itch • Hot water for laundry
Stasis Dermatitis[14]	• Pruritus, scaling, painless • Lower extremities, hemosiderin staining	• Lower extremity venous disease (*see page 67*) • Misdiagnosed as cellulitis	• Emollients: petrolatum, Lubriderm®, Eucerin®, Keri®, or Aquaphor® • Antibiotics only if bacterial infection
Varicella Zoster[15] **(Shingles)**	• Clusters of vesicles that appear along a dermatome with pain and itching	• Reactivation of the varicella zoster virus	• Antivirals (valacyclovir or acyclovir) • Medications for acute pain and postherpetic neuralgia

KEY POINTS

- Calciphylaxis is the calcification of small vessels in the body, which results in necrotic lesions. Localized wound care focuses on keeping the lesions dry by painting with povidone-iodine.
- Marjolin's ulcers reflect malignant changes in a chronic wound. Treatment focuses on tumor resection, lymph node dissection, or amputation.
- Lymphedema is a buildup of interstitial fluid and, without treatment, results in ulcerations. Exudate management is the primary goal of wound care.
- An enterocutaneous fistula is an opening between the gastrointestinal tract and skin. Effluent is the most distressing symptom. Manage effluent with dressings or wound pouches.
- Peristomal skin complications include mechanical trauma, infection, chemical irritants, diseases, and allergens. Management of the peristomal skin complication will vary based on the assessment of the complication.

References

1. Ely JW, Seabury M. The generalized rash: part I differential diagnosis. *Am Fam Physician*. 2010;81(6):726-734.
2. Page E. Description of skin lesions. June 2016. Merck Manual. Professional Version. Kenilworth, NJ;Merck and Co, Inc. 2018. https://www.merckmanuals.com/professional/dermatologic-disorders/approach-to-the-dermatologic-patient/description-of-skin-lesions Accessed May 2, 2018
3. Zhao CY, Murrell DF. Advances in understanding and managing bullous pemphigoid. F1000 Faculty Rev-1313. *F1000Res*. 2015;4:1-7. https://www.ncbi.nlm.nih.gov/pmc/articles/PMC4754018/ Accessed April 23, 2018.
4. Doggett SL, Dwyer DE, Penas PF, et al. Bed bugs: clinical relevance and control options. *Clin Microbiol Rev*. 2012 Jan;25(1):164-192.
5. Thomas S, Wrobel MJ, Brown J. Bedbugs: A primer for the health-system pharmacist. *Am J Health-Syst Pharm*. 2013; 70:126-30.
6. Kalra MG, Higgins KE, Kinney BS. Intertrigo and secondary skin infections. *Am Fam Physician*. 2014;89(7):569-573.
7. Gunderson C. Cellulitis: definition, etiology, and clinical features. *Am J Med* 2011;124(12):1113-1122.
8. Brasch J, Becker D, Aberer W, et al. Guideline contact dermatitis. *Allergo J Int*. 2014;23(4): 126-138.
9. Bryant RA. Types of skin damage and differential diagnosis. *Acute & Chronic Wounds: Current Management Concepts*. 4th ed. St Louis, MO: Elsevier/Mosby;2012:83-107.
10. Blume JE. Drug eruptions. Medscape. July 11, 2017 http://emedicine.medscape.com/article/1049474-overview. Accessed August 30, 2017.
11. Thomsen SF. Atopic dermatitis: natural history, diagnosis, and treatment. *ISRN Allergy*.2014:354250.
12. Satter EK. Folliculitis. Medscape. March 23, 2017 http://emedicine.medscape.com/article/1070456-overview Accessed August 30, 2017.
13. Chosidow O. Scabies. *N Eng J Med*. 2006;354:1718-1727.
14. Flugman SL. Stasis dermatitis treatment and management. Medscape April 17, 2017 http://emedicine.medscape.com/article/1084813-treatment#d11 Accessed August 30, 2017.
15. Cohen KR, Salbu RL, Frank J, et al. Presentation and management of herpes zoster (shingles) in the geriatric patient. *PT*. 2013;38(4):217-224,227.

OTHER THERAPIES

GOALS

- Discover emerging wound treatment options for pain and symptom management
- Compare evidence for topical medicated agents
- Learn recipes for common wound care preparations

LIDOCAINE TOPICAL GELS AND SOLUTIONS

Lidocaine is a local anesthetic available in both injectable and topical dosage forms. Injectable lidocaine is also used as an anti-arrhythmic agent. Lidocaine reduces peripheral nociceptor sensitization by blocking sodium ion channels to prevent initiation and conduction of nerve impulses producing anesthesia.[1,2] Topical lidocaine formulations may be used to manage wound pain associated with dressing changes, debridement, or other wound care procedures.[1-5] While the risk is low, even when applied to open wounds, there is some potential for systemic absorption of lidocaine from topical application.[2-4] Larger wounds, relative to the body size of the patient, may increase the risk of systemic absorption. Due to smaller body size, increased skin permeability, and changes in fat-water distribution of subcutaneous tissue, infants and small children also have an increased risk. Some topical lidocaine products have excipients that may cause burning or irritation (e.g., ethanol, benzyl alcohol, menthol, etc.). Oral topical lidocaine 2% solution, also known as viscous lidocaine, is designed specifically for mucous membrane use, potentially lessening the risk of systemic absorption. Although clinical literature is limited on the use of viscous lidocaine 2% for use in wound care, widespread availability, ease of use, clinical experience, and anecdotal evidence indicates it is the formulation of choice. Topical EMLA® (eutectic mixture of local anesthetics: lidocaine-prilocaine) cream has also been studied for painful wounds. EMLA® doses may range from 3g – 150g per application and is left in place for up to 60 minutes. Some patients report an uncomfortable burning sensation for several minutes after application.[5]

References
1. Lidocaine. Lexi-Drugs Online. Lexicomp. Wolters Kluwer; Hudson, OH. Accessed November 15, 2017.
2. Popescu A, Salcido R. Wound pain: a challenge for the patient and the wound care specialist. *Adv Skin Wound Care* 2004;17:14-22.
3. Pontani B, Feste M, Adams C, et al. Cross over clinical study of 47 patients with painful deep wounds showed use of a hydrogel containing 2% lidocaine HCl and collagen as contact layer was significant in alleviating dressing related pain. 23rd Clinical Symposium on Advances in Skin & Wound Care Oct 2008, no.30.
4. Evans E, Gray M. Do topical analgesics reduce pain associated with wound dressing changes or debridement of chronic wounds? *J Wound Ostomy Continence Nurs* 2005;32(5):287-290.
5. McDonald A, Lesage P. Palliative management of pressure ulcers and malignant wounds in patients with advanced illness. *J Palliat Med* 2005;9(2):285-295.

METRONIDAZOLE TOPICAL GEL, POWDER, CRUSHED TABLETS, SOLUTION

Metronidazole is likely the most studied medication used to control wound malodor. While applying crushed metronidazole tablets to malodorous wounds is a common practice in hospice care, the majority of published literature studies only metronidazole gel preparations or orally-administered metronidazole tablets.[1-6] Malodor in wounds is thought to be caused primarily by necrotic tissue and anaerobic bacteria.[1,2] Metronidazole's spectrum of anti-microbial activity covers protozoans and anaerobic Gram (+) and Gram (-) bacteria common in wounds (e.g., *Bacteroides, Fusobacterium, Peptostreptococci*).[1,7]

Metronidazole doesn't appear to be systemically absorbed at therapeutic levels from topical application; the anti-microbial benefit seems to be localized to the wound surface.[3] Lower dose oral metronidazole tablets, 250mg once or twice daily, can be considered for patients with wound odor that doesn't quickly respond to topical odor management with wound cleansers and anti-microbial dressings. Always review the patient's medication profile for potential drug interactions prior to initiating oral metronidazole.[2,3,6] Guide selection of the metronidazole dosage form for wound odor based on wound characteristics and patient need. Dry wound beds, though less likely to be malodorous, might benefit from a gel based dressing. Powdered metronidazole may be more appropriate for wounds with moderate to heavy exudate. Expect benefit from topical metronidazole within 2-3 days.[4]

Although metronidazole has been reported to control malodor in both malignant wounds and pressure injuries, topical metronidazole is a palliative symptom management technique not an attempt to eradicate infection in the wound. Refer to chapters on *Malignant Wounds* and *Pressure Injury Prevention and Treatment* for additional information on best practice for wound cleansing, appropriate debridement, and symptom management.

References

1. George R, Prasoona T, Kandasamy R, et al. Improving malodour management in advanced cancer: a 10-year retrospective study of topical, oral, and maintenance metronidazole. *BMJ Supp Palliat Care* 2017;7(3):286-291.
2. Watanabe K, Shimo A, Tsugawa K, et al. Safe and effective deodorization of malodorous fungating tumors using topical metronidazole 0.75% gel. *Support Care Cancer* 2016:24: 2583-2590.
3. Iida J, Kudo T, Shimada K, et al. Investigation of the safety of topical metronidazole from a pharmacokinetic perspective. *Biol Pharm Bull* 2013;36(1):89-95.
4. Ahkmetova A, Saliev T, Allan I, et al. Comprehensive review of topical odor-controlling treatment options for chronic wounds. J *Wound Ostomy Continence Nurs* 2016;43(6):598-609.
5. Paul J, Pieper B. Topical metronidazole for the treatment of wound odor: review of the literature. *Ostomy Wound Manage*. 2008;54(3):18-27.
6. Lyvers E, Elliott D. Topical metronidazole for odor control in pressure ulcers. *Cons Pharm* 2015;30(9):523-526.
7. Freeman C, Klutman N, Lamp K. Metronidazole: a therapeutic review and update. *Drugs* 1997;54(5):679-708

MORPHINE TOPICAL GEL

Topical morphine application to painful wounds may be appropriate for patients who have limited ulcer pain relief with systemic opioid therapy, or who develop intolerable opioid side effects such as excess sedation, severe constipation, or delirium. Topical opioid administration has been shown to provide analgesia for painful wounds if inflammation is present and the wound surface is visible.[1-3] Studies evaluating the benefit of topical morphine utilized a pharmacist-compounded mixture of morphine solution for injection and amorphous hydrogel.[1-3] Morphine gel seems to provide a varying duration of analgesia; application frequency varies by patient from 1-3 times per day.[1,3] Patients already taking systemic opioids for pain may have a diminished effect from topical application.[3] Wounds with intact skin and no inflammation are unlikely to respond to topical morphine gel. Topical opioid administration results in no systemic absorption and is not recommended for systemic pain relief.[4] For more information on topical morphine gel or solution, see Table 2 in this chapter.

References

1. Tran QNH, Fancher T. Achieving analgesia for painful ulcers using topically applied morphine gel. *J Support Oncol* 2007;5(6):289-293.
2. Zeppetella G, Joel SP, Ribeiro MDC. Stability of morphine sulphate and diamorphine hydrochloride in Intrasite gel. *Palliat Med* 2005;19:131-136.
3. Jacobson J. Topical opioids for pain. *Fast Facts and Concepts* FF185; 2015 https://www.mypcnow.org/blank-cu2j4 Accessed April 23, 2018.
4. Paice J, Von Roenn J, Hudgins J, et al. Morphine bioavailability from a topical gel formulation in volunteers. J Pain Symptom Manage 2008;35(3):314-320

PHENYTOIN TOPICAL GELS AND SOLUTIONS

Topical phenytoin (Dilantin®) use for acceleration of wound healing is based in the medication's ability to cause hyperplasia of gingival tissue. Phenytoin seems to stimulate collagen production and deposition in the wound and may decrease edema and bacterial load.[1] Wounds treated with topical phenytoin may have earlier healthy granulation tissue growth.[2] A small pilot study for treatment of chemotherapy-induced oral mucositis, results showed some improvement in pain and healing with use of topical phenytoin 0.5% oral rinse solution four times daily.[3] However, topical dressing of phenytoin in hydrogel demonstrated no benefit for diabetic foot ulcers in a randomized controlled trial.[4] In a study of patients with chronic venous wounds, daily application of a compounded topical phenytoin lotion, in conjunction with standard management practice for venous leg ulcers, resulted in a statistically significant faster rate of reduction in the size of the wound compared with placebo over an 8 week treatment study period.[2] Systematic review of the available literature seems to show a trend towards beneficial wound healing effects with the use of topical phenytoin. However, more data is needed before this treatment can be recommended.[1,5]

References

1. Shaw J, Hughes CM, Lagan KM, Bell PM. The clinical effect of topical phenytoin on wound healing: a systematic review. *Brit J Dermatol* 2007;157:997-1004.
2. Hokkam E, El-Labban G, Shams M, et al. Use of topical phenytoin for healing of chronic venous ulcerations. *Int J Surg* 2011;9(4):335-338.
3. Baharvand M, Sarrafi M, Alavi K, Jalali ME. Efficacy of topical phenytoin on chemotherapy-induced oral mucositis: a pilot study. *DARU* 2010;18(1):46-50.
4. Shaw J, Hughes CM, Lagan KM, Stevenson MR, Irwin CR, Bell PM. The effect of topical phenytoin on healing diabetic foot ulcers: a randomized controlled trial. *Diabet Med* 2011;28:1154-1157.
5. Xao X, Li H, Su H, Cai H, et al. Topical phenytoin for treating pressure ulcers. *Cochrane Db Syst Rev.* 2017;2:CD008251.

Table 1. Topical Medicated Agents for Skin and Wound Care[1]

Class	Medication (Brand)	Dosage Forms	Cost (Amt)*	Comments
Anesthetics	Lidocaine (Xylocaine®)	Cream, ointment, gel, solution	$ (100mL)	Viscous lidocaine 2% is recommended
	Lidocaine 2.5% - Prilocaine 2.5% (EMLA®)	Cream	$$ (30g)	Avoid application to open wounds
Antimicrobials	Bacitracin	Ointment	$ (15g)	Active against Gram+ bacilli. Risk of contact dermatitis with use developing over several days; anaphylaxis is rare but occurs rapidly after exposure
	Bacitracin & Polymyxin B (Polysporin®)	Ointment, powder	$ (15g)	
	Bacitracin, Polymyxin B, Neomycin (Neosporin®)	Ointment	$ (15g)	
	Cadexomer iodine (Iodosorb®)	Gel, ointment, tincture	$$$ (40g)	Broad spectrum germicidal against virus, bacteria, spores, fungi, protozoa
	Gentian violet (N/A)	Solution	$ (100mL)	Has antifungal and antimicrobial properties
	Honey – *Leptospermum* (Medihoney®)	Gel, paste	$$ (44g)	Broad spectrum antibacterial activity. Contraindicated if hypersensitivity to honey.
	Metronidazole 1% or 0.75% (Metrogel 1%®) (*1% is brand only*)	Gel	$$$ (0.75%) $$$$ (1%)	Powdered metronidazole tablets are more cost effective than commercial metronidazole gels but there is less evidence for efficacy.
	Mupirocin (Bactroban®, Centany®)	Cream, ointment	$$ (22g)	Active against MRSA, MSSA, *S. pyogenes*
	Silver sulfadiazine (Silvadene®)	Ointment	$ (25g)	Avoid use if sulfonamide allergy. Broad spectrum bactericidal activity.
Antifungals	Clotrimazole (Lotrimin®)	Cream, solution	$$ (30g)	Available with betamethasone (Lotrisone®)
	Ketoconazole (Extina 2%®, Xolegel 2%®)	Cream, foam, gel	$$ (30g)	Prescription gel & foam: $$$$
	Miconazole (Micatin®, Monostat®)	Cream, ointment, powder, spray	$$ (45g)	Available with zinc oxide (Baza AF®)
	Nystatin (Nystop®, Pedi-dri®)	Cream, ointment, powder	$$ (15g)	Available with triamcinolone (Mycolog-II®): $$$$
Barriers	Balsam Peru, Castor oil (Venelex®)	Ointment, spray	$$ (60g)	Not effective for debridement, mild bactericidal
	Vitamin A+D (Sween®, A+D®, Baza clear®)	Cream, ointment	$ (113g)	Do not use on severe burns or deep wounds
	Zinc oxide (Desitin®, Balmex®)	Cream, ointment, paste, powder	$ (113g)	Available with miconazole as Baza AF
Corticosteroids	Betamethasone (Celestone®, Diprolene®)	Cream, gel, lotion, ointment	$$$$ (50g)	For all topical corticosteroids: reassess use if no improvement within 14 days; corticosteroids can hinder wound healing and increase skin fragility Betamethasone+clotrimazole (Lotrisone®): $$$ Triamcinolone+nystatin (Mycolog-II®): $$$$
	Clobetasol (Clobex®, Temovate®)	Cream, foam, gel, lotion, ointment	$$$ (30g)	
	Fluocinonide (Lidex®, Vanos®)	Cream, gel, ointment	$$ (30g)	
	Fluocinolone (Derma-smoothe®)	Cream, oil, ointment	$$ (15g)	
	Hydrocortisone (Cortizone®, Cortaid®)	Cream, foam, gel, ointment	$ (15g)	
	Triamcinolone (Kenalog®, Triderm®)	Cream, lotion, ointment, spray	$$ (15g)	
Debriders	Collagenase (Santyl®)	Ointment	$$$$ (30g)	Will not affect healthy tissue, fat, fibrin, keratin, or muscle

Table 2. Recipes for Wound Care Preparations

Wound Prep	Components	Comments

Diluted hypochlorite solution (Dakin's®)[2]
• ¼ strength (0.125%)
• ½ strength (0.25%)
	• Household bleach (sodium hypochlorite 5.25%)
	    ○ ½ strength: 25 mL (1T+2 tsp)
	    ○ ¼ strength: 12.5 mL (2½ tsp)
	• ½ tsp baking soda
	• 32 oz boiled tap water*, cooled
	• 32 oz container, sterile
	Directions: Boil tap water, cool. Add ½ tsp of baking soda (buffering agent) and amount of bleach for desired strength of solution. Stir to dissolve and transfer to sterile container.
		• Dispose of any unused solution within 24 hours
		• Use only unscented, regular strength bleach (Clorox®)
		• Dakin's® solution is a commercially available product with published stability information; however, the stability and sterility of compounded hypochlorite solution cannot be guaranteed.
		• Short term use only (less than 14 days)

Acetic acid irrigation solution 0.25%[2,3]	• Distilled white vinegar ○ 0.25%: 50mL (3T+1 tsp) • 32 oz boiled tap water*, cooled • 32 oz container, sterile *Directions:* Boil tap water, cool. Add 50mL vinegar. Stir solution well and transfer to sterile container.	• Dispose of any unused solution within 24 hours • Acetic acid irrigation solution is a commercially available product with published stability information; however, the stability and sterility of compounded acetic acid solution cannot be guaranteed. • May have anti-*Pseudomonas* activity • Short term use only (less than 14 days)
Morphine in hydrogel[4]	• Morphine for injection (10mg/mL): 10mg (1mL) • Hydrogel (Intrasite®): 8g • Apply 5-10mL to wound and cover with dressing • May be applied 1 to 3 times per day	• Painful open wounds; no benefit if skin is intact and no systemic analgesic effect from topical application • Pharmacist-prepared compounded product is stable under controlled room temperature for 28 days.[5]
Morphine topical solution[6]	• Morphine for injection (10mg/mL): 20mg (2mL) • Normal saline: 8mL • Creates 0.2% morphine solution to be used as a topical spray for painful open wounds. *Alternate formulation*: Morphine 4% + Lidocaine 4% topical	• Painful open wounds • No benefit if skin is intact (stage 1 pressure injury) • No systemic analgesic effect • Pharmacist-prepared compounded product is stable under controlled room temperature for 14 days. • Larger volumes may be compounded
Metronidazole topical solution[7]	• Metronidazole (Flagyl®) tablet (500mg): 1000mg (2 tablets) • Normal saline: 100mL • Crush tablets and dissolve in 100mL of normal saline to create 1% solution. • Use as irrigation solution with dressing changes.	• Metronidazole topical solution may be prepared at bedside; discard any unused solution after each treatment • Metronidazole topical solution may be more effective to use for wounds with tunneling where powder from crushed tablets will not sufficiently reach

*Boil tap water 20 minutes and cool to room temperature. Prepare clean containers by boiling or sanitizing in dishwasher. Follow your organization's policy for clean vs sterile preparation.[2]

KEY POINTS

- Medicated topical gels and solutions are being investigated for their role in wound pain, symptom management and healing.
- Consider compounded topical medicated products for wound care when patient symptom management needs are refractory to commercially available products.
- Although commercially available, preparation of some wound care products can be done in the home when resources are scarce or access is difficult.

References

1. Lexi-Drugs Online. Lexicomp. Wolters Kluwer; Hudson, OH. Accessed November 15, 2017.
2. Brown P. Basics of wound management. In Brown P. *Quick Reference to Wound Care*. 4th ed. Burlington, MA: Jones & Bartlett Learning;2012:25-40.
3. Drosou A, Falabella A, Kirsner RS. Antiseptics on wounds: an area of controversy. *Wounds* 2003;15(6):149-166 http://www.woundsresearch.com/article/1586 Accessed April 23, 2018.
4. Tran QNH, Fancher T. Achieving analgesia for painful ulcers using topically applied morphine gel. *J Support Oncol* 2007;5(6):289-293.
5. Zeppetella G, Joel SP, Ribeiro MDC. Stability of morphine sulphate and diamorphine hydrochloride in Intrasite gel. *Palliat Med* 2005;19:131-136.
6. Jacobson J. Topical opioids for pain. *Fast Facts and Concepts* FF184; 2015 https://www.mypcnow.org/blank-cu2j4 Accessed April 23, 2018.
7. Zip CM. Innovative use of topical metronidazole. *Dermatol Clin* 2010;28(3):525-534.

WOUND CARE GLOSSARY

Term	Description
Ankle Brachial Index (ABI)	Method of assessing perfusion status, which determines if arterial disease is mild to severe. The Ankle Brachial Index is equal to the ankle systolic pressure divided by the brachial systolic pressure.
Abrasion	Wearing away of the skin through some mechanical process (friction or trauma).
Abscess	Accumulation of pus enclosed anywhere in the body.
Acute wound	Wound that heals timely and without complications. Can be created surgically or traumatically.
Antibiotic	*Pharmacologic agents* that destroy or inhibit bacteria. May be broad or narrow in spectrum of activity. May be used systemically and topically.
Antifungal	*Pharmacologic agents* that inhibit the growth of fungal infections. May be broad or narrow in spectrum of activity. May be used systemically and topically.
Antimicrobial	Any agent that destroys or inhibits the growth of microbes, including bacteria, fungi, viruses, or protozoa.
Antiseptic	*Chemical agents* that prevent, inhibit, or destroy microorganisms, including bacteria, viruses, fungi, and protozoa. Topical use only.
Autolysis	Disintegration or liquefaction of tissue or cells by the body's own mechanisms, such as leukocytes and enzymes.
Avoidable pressure injury	Pressure injury that results from facility failure to accurately assess patient risk factors and implement, monitor, and revise interventions based on the patient's assessment.
Bacterial burden	Total number of bacteria in a wound; may or may not cause a host response.
Bacteriostatic	Agent capable of inhibiting the growth of bacteria.
Biofilm	Polysaccharide matrix that microorganisms produce; highly resistant to antimicrobials. Must be removed by debridement.
Bioburden	Presence of microorganism on or in a wound. Continuum of bioburden ranges from contamination, colonization, critical colonization, biofilm and infection. Bioburden includes quantity of microorganism present, as well as their diversity, virulence, and interaction of the organism with each other and the body.
Blanching	Becoming white with the application of pressure.
Cachexia	Muscle wasting due to advanced disease.
Calciphylaxis	Calcification of small vessels in the body. Presents as painful mottling of the skin that deteriorates to necrosis.
Cellulitis	Inflammation of the tissues indicating a local infection; characterized by redness, edema, and tenderness.
Chronic wound	Wound that takes an extended period of time to heal, usually greater than four weeks, because of underlying factors, such as diabetes, pressure, poor nutrition, impaired circulation, or infection.
Clean wound bed	Granulating wound bed without devitalized tissue, signs and symptoms of infection, or excessive exudate.
Collagen	Main supportive protein of the skin.
Colonization	Presence of replicating bacteria that adhere to the wound bed but do not cause cellular damage to the host.
Complete decongestive therapy	Standard of care for lymphedema. Consists of manual lymph drainage, short stretch compression bandaging, lymphatic exercises, preventive skin care, and patient education.
Contact inhibition	Inhibition of cell activity (either locomotion or division) when in contact with neighboring cells.
Contamination	Non-replicating microorganisms on the wound surface without a host reaction. All open wounds are contaminated by normal skin flora.
Contraction	Myofibroblasts contract and bring wound edges closer together.
Critical colonization	Increasing bacterial load on a wound that is between the category of colonization and infection. The wound does not heal and may not display classic signs of infection.
Crusting	Technique used to assist with the adhesion of an appliance to denuded peristomal skin. To perform, apply light dusting of stomahesive powder, remove excess, pat with liquid barrier film and repeat x 2.
Dead space	Defect or cavity.
Debridement	Removal of foreign material, necrotic tissue, and slough from a wound until healthy tissue is exposed.
Decubitus	Latin word referring to the reclining position; misnomer for a pressure injury.

Term	Description
Demarcation	Line of separation between viable and nonviable tissue.
Denuded	Loss of epidermis.
Dermis	Inner layer of skin below the epidermis. Contains hair follicles and sweat glands.
Disinfectant	Topical liquid chemical that destroys or inhibits growth of microorganisms.
Dry desquamation	Pruritic, dry, flaking, or peeling skin in a patient with a history of radiation therapy to the affected area.
Enterocutaneous fistula	Opening between the gastrointestinal tract (stomach, small intestine, or large intestine) and the skin.
Enzymes	Biochemical substances capable of breaking down necrotic tissue.
Epibole	Rolled wound edge.
Epidermis	Outer most layer of skin.
Epithelialization	Process of the formation of new epithelial tissue (the outer-most layer of the skin).
Erosion	Loss of epidermis.
Erythema	Redness of the skin surface produced by vasodilation.
Eschar	Thick, leathery, black or brown crust; stable eschar is dry and firmly attached without exudate or fluctuance; unstable eschar is loosely adherent, wet, draining, erythematous, edematous, or fluctuant.
Excoriation	Linear scratches on the skin. NOT red or denuded.
Exudate	Accumulation of fluid in a wound; may contain serum, cellular debris, bacteria, and leukocytes.
Fistula	Abnormal passage from an internal organ to the body surface or between two internal organs.
Fluctuance	Moving in a wave-like manner suggesting the presence of fluid when alternating pressure is applied using two fingers.
Friction	Rubbing that causes mechanical trauma to the skin.
Full thickness	Tissue destruction extending through the dermis to involve subcutaneous level and possibly muscle, fascia, or bone.
Gelling fiber dressing	Absorbent dressing that forms a gel as it draws exudate and debris away from the wound bed.
Granulation	Formation of connective tissue and many new capillaries in a full thickness wound; typically appears as red and cobblestoned. Occurs only in a full thickness wound.
Granulation tissue	Pink to red, moist, fragile capillary tissue that fills a full thickness wound during the proliferative (cell division) phase of healing.
Granuloma	Nodules of immune cells. May appear as friable hypergranulation tissue.
Hydroconductive	Super absorbent dressing the draws exudate and debris away from the wound bed (e.g. Drawtex®).
Hydrophilic	Attracting moisture.
Hypergranulation tissue	Granulation tissue that forms above the level of the wound margins.
Hyperplasia	Enlargement of tissue because of increased cell reproduction.
Induration	Hardening of skin that would otherwise be soft.
Intermittent claudication	Pain with ambulation that resolves with rest.
Levine method	Preferred technique for obtaining a swab culture. To perform the Levine method, apply gentle pressure to the wound bed using a culture swab while rotating it over a one centimeter square area.
Lymphedema	Buildup of interstitial fluid as a result of a defect of the lymphatic system.
Maceration	Softening of tissue by soaking in fluids; looks like "dishpan hands."
Malnutrition	The lack of essential proteins and nutrients needed to flourish.
Device-related pressure injury	Pressure injuries to areas of the body excluding mucous membranes that are the result of medical devices.
Moist desquamation	Usually partial thickness tissue loss in a patient with a history of radiation therapy to the affected area. Can present as full thickness tissue loss if severe.
Moisture-associated skin damage	Skin inflammation and breakdown as a result of persistent contact to various sources of moisture, including urine, stool, perspiration, exudate, saliva, or ostomy effluent.
MRSA	Methicillin-Resistant *Staphylococcus aureus*.
MSSA	Methicillin-Susceptible *Staphylococcus aureus*.

Term	Description
Mucosal membrane pressure injury	Pressure injury present on the mucosal membrane as a result of a medical device.
Necrotic	Dead; avascular, nonviable.
Necrotic tissue	Dead, black or yellow tissue; when soft is referred to as slough, when hard is referred to as eschar.
Occlusive dressings	No liquids or gases can be transmitted through the dressing material.
Pallor	Lack of natural color; paleness.
Partial thickness	Wound that extends through the epidermis and may involve the dermis; heals by re-epithelialization.
Primary intention	Process of healing where wound edges are in close proximity to one another allowing the epithelial cells migrate from the wound edges and rapidly close the wound.
Purulent	Pus-like.
Pus	Thick fluid composed of leukocytes, bacteria, and cellular debris.
Pyoderma gangrenosum	Inflammatory autoimmune disease that results in painful ulcerations of the skin.
Radiation dermatitis	Localized skin reaction due to the administration of radiation therapy.
Regeneration	Process of replacing lost tissue with a replica of what was lost.
Reverse staging	Referring to healing pressure injuries in reverse order.
Sanguineous	Bloody exudate.
Scab	Crust of dried blood and serum.
Scar formation	Lost tissue is replaced with connective tissue that forms a scar over the wound bed.
Secondary intention	Process of healing when the wound edges are open and the defect is gradually filled in with scar tissue.
Semi-occlusive dressing	No liquids are transmitted through dressing naturally; variable level of gases can be transmitted through dressing material; most dressings are semi-occlusive.
Serous	Thin, watery exudate; clear to pale yellow.
Serosanguineous	Thin, red exudate; blood tinged serous fluid.
Shear	Sliding of skin over subcutaneous tissues and bones, causing a kink in cutaneous capillaries and ischemia.
Sinus tract	Course or pathway which can extend in any direction from the wound base; results in dead space with potential for abscess formation. Also referred to as tunneling.
Skin stripping/skin tears	Inadvertent removal of the epidermis, with or without the dermis, by mechanical means; precipitated by trauma, such as tape removal, bumping into furniture, or assisting with repositioning.
Slough	Deposits of dead white cells, dead bacteria, etc., in the wound bed, yellow in appearance; soft, moist, avascular/devitalized tissue; may be loose or firmly adherent.
Subcutaneous tissue	Layer of fat cells separated by connective tissue just below the dermis.
Toe brachial index (TBI)	Method of assessing the severity of arterial disease when the arteries of the ankle are noncompressible. The Toe Brachial Index is equal to the toe systolic pressure divided by the brachial systolic pressure.
Tunneling	Path of tissue destruction occurring in any direction from the surface or edge of a wound; results in dead space; involves small portion of wound edge; may be referred to as a sinus tract.
Unavoidable pressure injury	Development of a pressure injury despite accurately assessing patient risk factors and implementing, monitoring, and revising interventions based on the patient's assessment.
Undermine	Skin edges of a wound that have lost supporting tissue under intact skin.
VRE	Vancomycin-Resistant *Enterococcus*.
Wound bed preparation	Systematic approach of addressing wound bed characteristics that cause the healing process to stall.

References

1. Bryant RA, Nix DP, eds. *Acute & Chronic Wounds: Current Management Concepts.* 4th ed. St Louis, MO:Elsevier/Mosby;2012.
2. WOCN Glossary of Wound Care Terms. *Home Healthcare Now* 2003;21(8):512.
3. Zulkowski K. Wound terms and definitions. WCET J 2015;35(1): 22-27.

RESOURCE LIST

BOOKS

- Burghardt JC, Robinson JM, Tscheschlog BA, Bartelmo JM. *Wound Care Made Incredibly Visual.* 2nd ed. Philadelphia:Lippincott Williams Wilkins; 2012 [3rd edition available October 2018]
- Bryant RA, Nix DP, eds. *Acute & Chronic Wounds: Current Management Concepts.* 5th ed. St Louis, MO:Elsevier/Mosby; 2015
- Hess CT. *Clinical Guide to Skin and Wound Care.* 7th ed. Ambler, PA:Lippincottt, Williams & Wilkins; 2012

CERTIFICATION AGENCIES

- **American Board of Wound Management (CWS):** http://www.abwmcertified.org/
- **Wound, Ostomy and Continence Nursing Certification Board (CWOCN, CWON):** http://www.wocncb.org/
- **National Alliance of Wound Care and Ostomy (WCC):** http://www.nawccb.org/wound-care-certification

WOUND CARE JOURNALS

- **Advances in Skin and Wound Care:** http://journals.lww.com/aswcjournal
- **Advances in Wound Care:** http://www.liebertpub.com/overview/advances-in-wound-care/605/
- **Journal of the American College of Clinical Wound Specialists:** https://www.jaccws.org/
- **Journal of Wound Care:** http://www.journalofwoundcare.com
- **Journal of Wound, Ostomy & Continence Nursing:** https://journals.lww.com/jwocnonline
- **Ostomy Wound Management:** http://www.o-wm.com
- **Wound Care Advisor:** https://woundcareadvisor.com/
- **Wounds:** http://www.woundsresearch.com/node

MOBILE APPS

No charge; available for Android or Apple/iOS
- **3M Healthcare Pressure Ulcer Staging**
- **BSN Wounds App**
- **Choose a Dressing (interactive dressing selection)**
- **DermaRite (interactive dressing selection)**
- **Dressing Selection (Coloplast) (interactive dressing selection)**
- **Dressing Selection App (Acelity) (interactive dressing selection)**
- **Wound Central Mobile App**

ORGANIZATIONS

Association for the Advancement of Wound Care (AAWC): https://aawconline.memberclicks.net/
- A multidisciplinary organization with the mission of making wound care better for patients. It is a source of support, information, and education for patients, caregivers, researchers, educators, and practitioners across all settings, including acute, sub-acute, long-term care, and at home.

AHRQ: Agency for Healthcare Research and Quality: http://www.ahrq.gov/
- AHRQ, a division of the U.S. Department of Health & Human Services, aims to improve the quality, safety, efficiency, and effectiveness of healthcare for all Americans.

BioTherapeutics, Education and Research Foundation (BTER): http://www.bterfoundation.org
- A non-profit organization specializing in public support and professional education in biotherapeutic medicine. Biotherapy is the use of live animals to aid in the diagnosis or treatment of illness.

Hope of Healing Foundation: http://hopeofhealing.org
- Organization founded by physicians to provide community outreach and wound care strategies to prevent amputation.

NPUAP-National Pressure Ulcer Advisory Panel: http://www.npuap.org/
- American National Pressure Ulcer Advisory Panel: An independent, non-profit, professional organization promoting evidence-based care for pressure injuries.

TOOLS

- **Braden Risk Assessment Scale:** Used to assess a patient's risk of developing a pressure injury and the degree of risk. See website for additional information: http://www.bradenscale.com/
- **FRAIL Palliative Wound Care Palliative Wound Care and Healing Probability Assessment Tool:** Used to assess the potential for wound healing. Available at: http://www.frailcare.org/images/Palliative%20Wound%20Care.pdf
- **Hunters Hill Marie Curie Centre Pressure Ulcer Risk Assessment:** Pressure injury risk assessment specific to the palliative care population. Available at: https://nursekey.com/palliative-wound-care/
- **Nutritional Screening Tools:**
  - Mini Nutritional Assessment-Short Form
    http://www.mna-elderly.com/forms/mna_guide_english_sf.pdf
  - Malnutrition Universal Screening Tool
    http://www.bapen.org.uk/pdfs/must/must_full.pdf
  - Short Nutritional Assessment Questionnaire
    http://www.fightmalnutrition.eu/fight-malnutrition/screening-tools/snaq-tools-in-english/
- **Pressure Ulcer Scale for Healing (PUSH):** Used to assess improvement or deterioration of pressure injuries. Available at: http://www.npuap.org/wp-content/uploads/2012/02/push3.pdf
- **Wound, Ostomy, Continence Nurses Society™ Support Surface Algorithm:** An evidence-based algorithm for support surface selection. Available at: http://algorithm.wocn.org/#home

WEBSITES

International Skin Tear Advisory Panel: http://www.skintears.org/
- Online resource for the assessment, prevention, and management of skin tears.

Ostomy Wound Management: http://www.o-wm.com/home
- Journal for health care professionals addressing ostomy, wound, incontinence, skin, and nutritional issues. Includes Wounds 360 online wound care products resource.

World Council of Enterostomal Therapists: http://www.wcetn.org/
- Association for nurses involved in ostomy, wound, and continence care.

Wound Care Advisor: http://woundcareadvisor.com/
- Official online journal of National Alliance of Wound Care (NAWC) covering wound, skin, and ostomy management.

Wound Ostomy and Continence Nurses Society: http://www.wocn.org/
- Nursing society supporting educational, clinical, and research opportunities. *Photography in Wound Documentation: Fact Sheet* available via the WOCN website.

WoundSource.com: http://www.woundsource.com/
- Provides wound care professionals clinically-reviewed wound care supply information. Includes over 1,000 products manufactured by over 150 wound care companies.

WorldWideWounds.com: http://www.worldwidewounds.com/
- Web-based wound care journal covering dressing materials and wound management topics.

Wounds360bg.com: http://www.wounds360bg.com
- Provides product information for wound care clinicians, such as support surfaces, compression, and offloading devices.

ADDITIONAL AGENCIES/RESOURCES

- **Academy of Nutrition and Dietetics:** http://www.eatright.org/
- **American Academy of Dermatology:** https://www.aad.org/
- **American Academy of Wound Management:** http://www.abwmcertified.org/
- **American College of Foot and Ankle Surgeons:** http://www.acfas.org/
- **American College of Hyperbaric Medicine:** http://www.achm.org/
- **American Diabetes Association:** http://www.diabetes.org/
- **American Physical Therapy Association:** https://www.apta.org/
- **American Podiatric Medical Association:** https://www.apma.org/
- **American Professional Wound Care Association:** http://www.apwca.org/
- **American Venous Forum:** http://veinforum.org/
- **Association for the Advancement of Wound Care:** http://aawconline.org/
- **Dermatology Nurses Association:** http://www.dnanurse.org/
- **National Association for Support of Long Term Care:** https://www.nasl.org/eweb/startpage.aspx
- **Society for Vascular Medicine:** http://www.vascularmed.org/
- **Society for Vascular Surgery:** https://vascular.org/
- **Wound Healing Society:** http://woundheal.org/

NOTES

NOTES

INDEX

i

Made in the USA
Middletown, DE
10 January 2020